The Bloggers Diet

Journal your way to the S.E.X.Y. you!

Nakisha Guzman

ISBN: 978-0-6152-1506-8

Always consult your medical professional before starting any of the suggestions in this book.
The author and publisher will not be responsible for any liability, loss, or risk, personal or otherwise in relation to applicable use of this book.

If you prefer to blog instead of journaling in this book, you can visit our website at www.bloggersdiet.com. You can sign up, create an account and begin blogging (online journal) about your journey and finally, your success story. Visit often for frequent updates and awesome tools. You can also receive personalized consults & online fitness training from Nakisha by visiting www.nakishaguzman.com.

To help you have a flourishing inner and outer body so that life is enjoyed and not endured.

Contents

Introduction

I am glad that you are reading this book. Your time has arrived. You no longer have to be a slave to food. You will become the master of your mind. If you can control your thinking, you can control the urge to splurge. There is a military saying that goes, "If you don't mind, it doesn't matter." Basically, what this statement is saying is mind over matter. The matter for you could be lack of exercise, junk food eating, gorging and bingeing, or just plain lack of knowledge. No more excuses, no more failure. I provide you with the tools; all you have to do is use them. Are you ready to be free?

I know some of the contents will be considered unconventional for many, but it is statistically apparent that conventional plans are not working for Americans today.

You can use this book in many ways. The main goals are to get you feeling and looking S.E.X.Y. Sexy, not in the way the media has taught us to view and label sexy, but my personal vision of S.E.X.Y.: A slimmer, energetic, eXuberant and youthful you!

I speak candidly and I get right to the point. I have counseled many individuals on eating the foods that strengthen the body, and on the importance of getting fit daily. What I have noticed is that with all the diet plans available, very few actually read the book from cover to cover. They all want the fix and they want it fast. Therefore, I decided to give it to you all up front, and if and when you decide to dive in for more details, you can flip to the back rooms.

This book is simple and the principles are easy when

followed correctly. I've designed the book into different rooms to assist you at whatever stage you are at when you begin reading.

Who is Nakisha Guzman?

I am no stranger to hardcore fitness. I was a Sergeant in the U.S. Army, married and had only one child during this time. I enjoyed the look that fitness gave me but paid little to no attention to my diet. I believe that my young age and busy lifestyle allowed me to stay 'slim' without focusing on the nutrients of food. However, after leaving the military, having four children, and becoming a stellar baker, I found myself staring at 160 lbs on a 5' 2" frame. I decided enough was enough after seeing some pictures from one of our home parties. It was during this moment that I re-visited my health book that I began writing back in 2003. Armed with determination and drive, I not only transformed my book but my body as well. In just a few short months of beginning as my personal test person, I went from 160 lbs to 140 lbs and lost inches all over (and continued to lose weight & inches). While on this journey, I struggled with not being able to connect with other likeminded individuals. I was unable to express my inner struggles and receive feedback. It was from this disconnect that The Bloggers Diet was born.

I have a passion for food, fitness and enjoying life. My mission is to connect people so that fitness & nutrition become a way of life not just a '3 month plan'. I am a Certified Personal Trainer and I have assisted many individuals with understanding what foods to eat, teaching them how foods affect the body, and laying out simple workout routines to help folks get moving in the right direction.

I am a devout follower of Christ, wife of 12 years, and mother to 4 beautiful girls.

Now that you know a little bit about me, let us jump into how the Bloggers Diet will work for you!

Here Is How It Works

If you have spent a lifetime or long time eating junky foods (you know what junky foods are), and not exercising consistently, then the 180-degree section is where you'll need to begin. Your progression will lead you into the next section. The past is behind you and your future looks fabulous!

If you eat relatively well; meaning you stay clear of greasy burgers, French fries, fried food, any items that contain partially hydrogenated oils, but want to lose a few extra pounds, or are ready to go to the next level in nutrition, you begin in the Boot Camp Body section.

In the section titled, Be Fit Not Fake, I give you the entire rundown of the whys & hows of food, supplements, and fitness.

In the last section, Make It Happen, you will find a surplus of additional tools and tips that will assist you in making the Bloggers Diet happen for you.

Find your section and get S.E.X.Y.

Results That Last

First 60 days plan

	STARTING	ENDING
WEIGHT	150	133
ABDOMEN	37.5 INCHES	31.5 INCHES
HIPS	44.50 INCHES	41.5 INCHES
BODY FAT	29.4	19.5

A Moment To Reflect

When you break goals into increments and start controlling your time, things begin to happen. Zig Ziglar

Teach us how short our lives really are so that we may be wise. Psalm 90:12 (NCV)

Room 1
180 DEGREES

Welcome to the making of the S.E.X.Y. you. This room will give you the tools you need to make small but effective changes to your current eating patterns, helping you to achieve very successful results. When you complete this room, you will be slimmer, have more energy, and feel such glee, as you will have conquered the SAD (standard American diet) lifestyle of overeating, emotional eating, and no exercise.

180 degrees is a journal mapping my return to good health and fitness, after being on a 2-year hiatus. After giving birth to two more children back to back, I lost my eating healthy notion, which had defined me in the preceding years.

I was going nowhere fast, and I decided enough was enough. I was tired of not fitting into my clothes, I was tired of sucking my belly in, and I was tired of feeling burned down. The next 30 days were the jumpstart I needed to get back to core healthiness.

Here is how this will work for you. I have provided my blog entries and fitness regimen for this time frame. You will use this as motivation for your journey. I have also created an area where you can record your day in the same manner as I did. Each tool goes hand in hand. You will change your eating, you will exercise, and you will release your feelings by journaling. If possible, I would like you to incorporate a partner, or better yet, create a neighborhood Bloggers Diet group. This partner or group will be very helpful; when you are feeling a little weak, someone from your group can give the encouragement and accountability that you need to pull through. Life should be done together! We were created for relationships. If you find (like I did) that your immediate friends are not interested in being healthy in order to live a long, effective life; don't worry, just go to www.bloggersdiet.com, you can create your own personalized Bloggers Diet page, and connect with an e-partner to walk alongside your journey to the S.E.X.Y. you or for a personalized plan visit www.nakishaguzman.com.

STEPS TO SUCCESS

Now that you understand the concept; you will find below some of the recommended tools for the journey.

First, you will need to make yourself accountable. If you are truly ready to take your life back, then take this simple but priceless step. When we put things to writing and make them binding, it opens the door to commitment. With commitment and dedication, you can achieve the desired results.

THE COMMITMENT LETTER

I, _____, agree to begin my training on this day, _____,

➢ I agree to put forth all my efforts into attaining tons of energy, a healthy mind and a totally fit body.
➢ I will make every effort to be tightened, toned, and terrific.
➢ I will not allow food to run me; I will run it because I am in charge.
➢ I realize that my body is a wonderfully made temple that I must maintain with high regard and high standards.
➢ I will not allow non health-conscious individuals to discourage me. I deserve to be and feel my best at all times.
➢ I choose NOW to leave both laziness and excessive food consumption behind.
➢ I am creating a new way that will keep me healthy for years to come.
➢ I have told_____about my journey because they are a part of my support system, and they agree to encourage me to drive forward.

Nothing can stop me now but myself, and I have the ability to control and change me.

Signature_____
Date_____

Our planet has gone from naturally clean foods and water to packaged foods and bottled everything. How can we fill these nutritional gaps? Supplementation is the answer. Many nutrients are found in whole foods like vegetables, whole grains and fruits, but very few people eat the correct amount in the run of a busy day.

Below, you will find supplements that will assist you in feeling great while you begin this process.

SUPPLEMENTS THAT MAKE YOU FEEL GREAT

- Multi-Vitamin (for overall balance and health)
- B100 (for energy)
- EFA (Essential Fatty Acids) visit your local health food store and speak with a rep about any of these products.
- CLA (Conjugated Linoleic Acid)
- Green Tea and Black Tea
-

You can visit your local health food store to find these products.

THE GROCERY LIST

Here is an ideal grocery shopping list. Remember, in this room, we are gradually shifting our connection with junk food, and re-training our palates to desire healthier foods.

Meats, Fish, and Poultry:
Lean ground beef (limit to once or twice a month, if at all)
Lean beef steak cuts (limit to once or twice a month, if at all)
Luncheon meats 95% or better lean (no nitrates)
Lean chicken (breast and skinless the best)
Seafood (salmon, tilapia, and so forth)

Turkey bacon
Eggs, Dairy, and Fats:
Low fat cheeses
100% Whole grain bread
Butter (not margarine)
Olive oil (extra virgin and cold pressed)
Eggs (try vegetarian fed)
Non-fat milk or soy milk
Fruits and Vegetables:
All vegetables (fresh or frozen over canned)
Romaine, leaf and spinach lettuce (not iceberg)
Cucumbers, celery, peppers, onions, tomatoes, etc.
All berries
Grapefruit
Cherries
Limes and lemons
Pineapples
Apples
Legumes
Chick Peas (high in fiber)
Black Beans (high in fiber)
Lentils (high in fiber)
Nuts and Seeds:
Raw Almonds
Pumpkin Seeds
Sunflower Seeds
Pistachios

Condiments, Sweeteners, Seasonings:

Stevia Plus (found at most health food stores)

Iodized sea salt (use sparingly)

You select seasonings, but limit salt & sugar added blends

Drinks:

Club soda

Sparkling water

Water, water, water

Limit coffee (one a day, moving to one a week, to none)

Green and Black Tea (plain or sweeten with Stevia or 1 tsp of honey and lemon)

Miscellaneous:

Regular oatmeal

Whole wheat rice and pasta

Mustard and Dijon

Salsa

Vinegars

All seasonings (limit or avoid excess salt)

Broths

Olive oil

Trans fat-free healthy mayonnaise

Healthy snacks for home or carry

Seeds

Nuts

Fresh fruit

Carrot sticks

Apples –(green is best)
Grapes
All berries and melons
Frozen popsicles
Dried fruit
Boiled eggs
Yogurts
Raisins
Pineapples

THE PLAN

Step 1: Find a partner, group, e-partner or a combination. △

Step 2: Sign and post your commitment letter around the home, desk and car. △

Step 3: Remove any food from your home that contains partially hydrogenated oils (read ingredients labels), high fructose corn syrup, and definitely no sodas (of any type).△

Step 3: Build meals based on food items from the aforementioned grocery list. You can also preview a week of my journaling, and mimic the meals! △

Step 4: Incorporate exercise. △

Step 5: Stay connected with others, get all the motivation you desire from www.bloggersdiet.com, and enjoy the journey that will lead you to the S.E.X.Y. you!

THE EXTRAS FOR SUCCESS

✓ Stay clear of fast food restaurants. If you are in a crunch, never go hungry; simply choose chicken over burgers, grilled or baked over fried, no mayo, extra lettuce & tomato, no fries, no soda… drink water! If you prepare your healthy life-giving cuisines on Sunday, then you eliminate the likelihood of entertaining fast food.

✓ Daily, drink a minimum of 64 oz of water and consume green tea as often as possible…no sugar please!

Inspire Me: Every journey begins with the first step. Make the move today.

Tell fat goodbye…Your new journey begins NOW!

Day 1 – Monday, July 9th

Today was an easy day. My motivation meter was on a high, and I felt like I could conquer any battle. I haven't gone to the grocery store yet, so finding snack options was difficult. Late in the evening, I had a hunger attack. I was watching TV and suddenly I wanted cookies. Why? I don't know, maybe I was sleepy. I went downstairs and announced to one of my daughters and my husband that I was hungry and was making a salad. They smiled. My husband, of course, was smiling because he knew the struggle that I was going through. Today was a great day.

Today I ate:

Breakfast
One package of oatmeal
Supplements: Multi-vitamin, EFA (essential fatty acids), and B-100
Drinks: green tea with Xylitol, and 16.9 oz of water

Lunch
Chicken salad with grilled chicken, low fat balsamic vinaigrette, lettuce, tomatoes, onions, corn and black beans
Black coffee - no sugar, no cream
20 oz water

Dinner
Black beans, ½ cup to 1 cup, seasoned with oregano, garlic, onion, and olive oil
2- Baked chicken legs seasoned with the above ingredients
20 oz water

Evening Snack

Green leaf lettuce salad with tomatoes, onions, banana peppers, and 1 tablespoon of Roka Bleu cheese

For Fitness

Cardio - 30 minutes on the treadmill at incline 2.0 to 3.0 in 6-minute intervals.

Strength - 3 sets of 12 - bicep curls, lateral raises, upright rows, triceps kickbacks, overhead triceps work, bicep curls again, and 15 (knee) pushups.

Abs - 10 minutes of crunches and bicycles.

Now it's your turn. Begin the diet that will give you the results you want to see. Begin the diet that will become a way of life. not just a 30-day program.

Day 1-_____

Journal Entry

_____
_____
_____
_____
_____
_____
_____
_____
_____
_____
_____
_____
_____
_____

Today I ate:

Breakfast

_____

_____

_____

_____

_____

_____

_____

_____

_____

Lunch

_____

_____

_____

_____

_____

_____

_____

_____

_____

Dinner

_____

_____

_____

_____

_____

_____

_____

_____

Snack (max 2 a day)

For Fitness

Cardio -

Strength -

Abs -

Day 2 – Tuesday, July 10th

Wow, what a day. I got lots of housework done. I felt super. I can feel myself returning to a lifestyle that is suited for victory. If I can accomplish mind control and self-control over food, then I can do anything. Food can be addictive, especially if you find yourself home alone, and not being productive in your purpose in life. Even when you choose not to enjoy a hobby for yourself, you will find yourself unbalanced, and become easily frustrated. I'm glad I am back on the road to being balanced. I have four daughters who are watching me, and I must set an example of how to be a strong women.

Today I ate:

Breakfast
One package of oatmeal
Supplements: Multi-vitamin, EFA (essential fatty acids), and B-100
Drinks: green tea with Xylitol, and 16.9 oz of water

Lunch
Turkey sandwich with mustard, green leaf lettuce, tomato slices, 1 slice provolone cheese, 2 slices of low-carb bread
1 medium green apple
20 oz water

Dinner
Black beans, ½ cup to 1 cup, seasoned with oregano, garlic, onion, and olive oil.
2 baked chicken legs seasoned with the above ingredients.
20 oz water

Evening Snack
10 organic animal crackers (this is one serving)

For Fitness
Cardio - 40 minutes on the treadmill at incline 2.0 to 3.0 in6 minute intervals.
Strength - 3 sets of 12 - machine leg press (110lb), 3 sets of 12 inner thigh and outer thigh gym machine (abductor/abduction), and 3 sets of 12 calf raises
Abs -10 minutes of crunches and bicycles

It's Your Turn...

Day 2-_____

Journal Entry

_____
_____
_____
_____
_____
_____
_____
_____
_____
_____
_____
_____
_____

Today I ate:

Breakfast

_____
_____
_____
_____
_____
_____
_____
_____
_____

Lunch

_____
_____
_____
_____

_____

_____

_____

_____

_____

Dinner

_____

_____

_____

_____

_____

_____

_____

Snack (max 2 a day)

_____

_____

_____

For Fitness
Cardio -

_____

_____

Strength -

_____

_____

_____

_____

_____

Abs -

_____

_____

Day 3 – Wednesday, July 11th

Today was super hectic. Not only did I wake up late with 4 kids to get to various locations around the same time, but there was also a storm. Currently, my youngest two are 23 months old and 8 months old, and my 7-year-old has special needs. So needless to say, jumping in and out of the car with those three was a little challenging. I got my 10-year-old off to her camp first, since she had to be there by 8:45 or she would have missed the ride to the movies. My 7-year-old is in a special needs camp style program offered by the YMCA. She has to be there at 8:30 because at 9:00 they leave for the pool. I got there at 9:03... they were already in the pool. Normally, this would not be a problem, but I didn't bring the baby in the carry as she was on my hip. My toddler is eager to run the minute I let loose of her hand, and I had to get my 7-year-old undressed (she wears a hearing device that can't get wet) while holding the baby on my knee, and constantly in a pleasant voice reminding my toddler to wait, don't move, yes look at the pretty blue water. Finally someone from her class saw her and they took over. I got the babies to their mother's day out program almost 50 minutes late. However, now I was kid free for at least an hour and a half. Instead of chilling, I ran to the library and spent too much time there only to find myself rushing back to the YMCA for a brief cardio workout, and then I had to run up and get my 7-year-old. The remainder of the day was equally as busy, but it was on my schedule as busy, so that wasn't so bad. Oh, and by the way, did I happen to mention that my cycle started today?

Today I ate:

Breakfast
One package of oatmeal
Supplements: Multi-vitamin, EFA (essential fatty acids), and B-100
Drinks: green tea with Xylitol, and 16.9 oz of water

Lunch
Turkey sandwich with mustard, green leaf lettuce, tomato slices, 1 slice provolone cheese, 2 slices of low-carb bread.
1 medium green apple
20 oz water

Dinner
1 natural burger on 2 slices of low-carb bread with mustard, lettuce, tomato, and onion.
Green leaf lettuce salad with 1 tablespoon of corn, 1 tablespoon of black olives, onion slices, tomato slices, and I tablespoon of Roka Bleu cheese dressing.
20 oz water

Evening Snack
10 Pretzels and 16.9 oz water

For Fitness
Cardio - 20 minutes on elliptical
Strength - 3 sets of 12 - bicep curls, lateral raises, upright rows, triceps kickbacks, overhead triceps work, bicep curls again, and 15 (knee) pushups.
Abs -10 minutes of crunches and bicycles

It's Your Turn...

Day 3-_____

Journal Entry

_____
_____
_____
_____
_____
_____
_____
_____
_____
_____
_____
_____

Today I ate:

Breakfast

_____
_____
_____
_____
_____
_____
_____
_____

Lunch

_____

_____

_____

_____

_____

_____

_____

_____

_____

Dinner

_____

_____

_____

_____

_____

_____

_____

Snack (max 2 a day)

_____

_____

_____

For Fitness
Cardio -

_____

_____

Strength -

_____

_____

_____

_____
_____
_____

Abs -

_____
_____

Day 4 – Thursday, July 12th

Great start to my morning. No rush. Boo was able to help so I didn't have to take all the kids to drop my 7-year-old off at camp. I handled some errands this morning and spent most of the day gathering my thoughts. I really needed to reorganize my workspace, and I needed to balance all the ideas in my head. I'm passionate about writing, although I rarely find as much time as I would like to devote to doing it. I realize this is my season of growth, and a young season of parenting, so I am ok with my progress. I worked out in the evening today. I felt really good when I returned home, although it was a much later dinner than I would have liked (10:00 pm). Yes, I know that is very bad. I worked out at about 7:30 pm. I wouldn't say that I had a hard time going to sleep, but I did think a little before I went off to dream land. Normally, I hit the pillow and it's lights out!

Today I ate:

Breakfast
One package of oatmeal
Supplements: Multi-vitamin, EFA (essential fatty acids), and B-100
Drinks: green tea with Xylitol, and 16.9 oz of water

Lunch

Turkey sandwich with mustard, green leaf lettuce, tomato slices, 1 slice provolone cheese, 2 slices of low-carb bread.
1 medium green apple
20 oz water

Dinner
 6 oz sirloin steak
Salad with tomatoes, onions, carrots, and balsamic vinaigrette.
20 oz water

Evening Snack
None

For Fitness
Cardio - 20 minutes on treadmill and 20 minutes on elliptical.
Strength - 3 sets of 12 - machine leg press (110lb), 3 sets of 12 inner thigh and outer thigh gym machine (abductor/abduction), and 3 sets of 12 calf raises
Abs -10 minutes of crunches and bicycles.

It's Your Turn...

Day 4-_____

Journal Entry

_____
_____
_____
_____
_____
_____
_____
_____

_____

_____

_____

_____

_____

_____

Today I ate:

<u>Breakfast</u>

_____

_____

_____

_____

_____

_____

_____

_____

_____

<u>Lunch</u>

_____

_____

_____

_____

_____

_____

_____

_____

_____

<u>Dinner</u>

_____

_____

_____
_____
_____
_____
_____
_____
_____
_____

Snack (max 2 a day)

_____
_____
_____
_____

For Fitness
Cardio -

_____
_____

Strength -

_____
_____
_____
_____
_____
_____

Abs -

_____
_____

Day 5 – Friday, July 13th

Why was my toddler crying at 4:30 in the morning? I decided to just stay up. I mean, I have a lot that I could research in the quiet time of the morning. My clock was set for 6:00 am and it was almost 5:00 before she settled.

Today I ate:

Breakfast

One package of oatmeal
Supplements: Multi-vitamin, EFA (essential fatty acids), and B-100
Drinks: green tea with Xylitol, and 16.9 oz of water

Lunch

Turkey sandwich with mustard, green leaf lettuce, tomato slices, 1 slice provolone cheese, 2 slices of low-carb bread.
1 medium green apple
20 oz water

Dinner

1 natural burger on 2 slices of low-carb bread with mustard, lettuce, tomato, and onion.
Green leaf lettuce salad with 1 tablespoon of corn, 1 tablespoon of black olives, onion slices, tomato slices, and I tablespoon of Roka Bleu cheese dressing.
20 oz water

Evening Snack

10 Pretzels and 16.9 oz water

For Fitness

Cardio -20 minutes on elliptical.
Strength - 3 sets of 12 - bicep curls, lateral raises, upright rows, triceps kickbacks, overhead triceps work, bicep curls again, and 15 (knee) pushups.
Abs -10 minutes of crunches and bicycles.

It's Your Turn...

Day 5-_____

Journal Entry

_____
_____
_____
_____
_____
_____
_____
_____
_____
_____
_____
_____
_____

Today I ate:

Breakfast

_____
_____
_____
_____
_____
_____
_____
_____

Lunch

_____

_____

_____

_____

_____

_____

_____

_____

Dinner

_____

_____

_____

_____

_____

_____

_____

Snack (max 2 a day)

_____

_____

_____

For Fitness
Cardio -

_____

Strength -

_____

_____

_____

_____

_____

Abs -

_____

_____

Day 6 – Saturday, July 14th

Today was extremely busy. I had an 8:30 am hair appointment and today was Grandma's birthday party. She turned 89. Of course, we were rushing and the day flew by. I was very tired today, although I am looking forward to entering a fitness competition. I have to get my info by Sunday. At the party, they served pizza and cupcakes. I didn't have any! Yah for me. My cheat day is Sunday!

Today I ate:

Breakfast
One package of oatmeal
Supplements: Multi-vitamin, EFA (essential fatty acids), and B-100
Drinks: green tea with Xylitol, and 16.9 oz of water

Lunch
Chicken salad from Sonic, with Italian dressing (no croutons).
20 oz water

Dinner
Grilled chicken breast
Corn

20 oz water

Evening Snack
10 animal cookies and 16.9 oz water

For Fitness
Cardio - 30 minutes jogging and jumping rope.

It's Your Turn...

Day 6-_____

Journal Entry

_____
_____
_____
_____
_____
_____
_____
_____
_____
_____
_____
_____
_____
_____

Today I ate:

Breakfast

_____
_____

_____
_____
_____
_____
_____
_____
_____

Lunch

_____
_____
_____
_____
_____
_____
_____

Dinner

_____
_____
_____
_____
_____
_____
_____

Snack (max 2 a day)

_____
_____
_____

For Fitness
Cardio -

Strength -

Abs -

Day 7 – Sunday, July 15th

Wow, I'm feeling great. I have conquered my first week. There are still areas of my eating that I need to tighten up. I need to cut the pretzels & animal crackers, but I'm on my way. Today is our family party for Uncle & Trin. I cooked chicken, black beans, brown rice, and cornbread. We had a really good time and it was a nice family moment. Today was my cheat day, and I had one ice-cream cup cake and cornbread with my meal.

Today I ate:

Breakfast
One package of oatmeal
Supplements: Multi-vitamin, EFA (essential fatty acids), and B-100

Drinks: green tea with Xylitol, and 16.9 oz of water

Lunch
Jersey Mike's -sub in a tub -lettuce, tomato, onions, ham, turkey, provolone, oregano, salt & pepper, oil & vinegar.
20 oz water

Dinner
Grilled chicken drumsticks - 2 pieces.
Corn -1/3 cup
Black beans -1 cup
Brown rice -½ cup
20 oz water

Evening Snack
1-ice cream cupcake and 16.9 oz water

For Fitness
None

It's Your Turn...

Day 7-_____

Journal Entry
_____
_____
_____
_____
_____
_____
_____
_____

_____

_____

_____

_____

_____

_____

Today I ate:

Breakfast

_____

_____

_____

_____

_____

_____

_____

_____

_____

Lunch

_____

_____

_____

_____

_____

_____

_____

_____

_____

Dinner

_____

_____

_____
_____
_____
_____
_____
_____
_____

Snack (max 2 a day)

_____
_____
_____

For Fitness
Cardio -

_____
_____

Strength -

_____
_____
_____
_____
_____

Abs -

_____
_____

Day 8 – Monday, July 16th

Although I am very blessed to be alive & breathing, my morning started off very sour. I got into a huge spat with my close friend/business partner. This caused me to run late getting out of the house. I did have an awesome workout, and was able to clear out a lot of things in my head pertaining to my home, my heart, and my family.

Today I ate:

Breakfast
One package of oatmeal
Supplements: Multi-vitamin, EFA (essential fatty acids), and B-100
Drinks: green tea with Xylitol, and 16.9 oz of water

Lunch
½ Toasted chicken sandwich from Sonic.
20 oz water

Dinner
Grilled chicken drumsticks - 2 pieces.
Corn -½ cup
Black Beans -1 cup
20 oz water

Evening Snack
10 animal crackers 16.9 oz water

For Fitness
Cardio -35 minutes on the elliptical
Lower – Strength -3 sets of 12 -machine leg press (110lb), 3 sets of 12 inner thigh and outer thigh gym machine (abductor/abduction), and 3 sets of 12 calve raises.
Abs -10 minutes of crunches and bicycles

It's Your Turn...

Day 8-_____

Journal Entry

_____
_____
_____
_____
_____
_____
_____
_____
_____
_____
_____
_____
_____

Today I ate:

Breakfast

_____
_____
_____
_____
_____
_____
_____
_____

Lunch

_____

_____
_____
_____
_____
_____
_____
_____
_____

Dinner

_____
_____
_____
_____
_____
_____
_____

Snack (max 2 a day)

_____
_____
_____

For Fitness
Cardio -

_____
_____

Strength -

_____
_____
_____

_____

_____

_____

Abs -

_____

_____

Day 9 – Tuesday, July 17th

Wow, today started off well but when I arrived at the gym, Trinity, my 23-month-old, burst into tears. She did not want to go into the child care area. Feeling bad and upset, I decided to leave and come back home. Tori, my oldest, was a little disappointed, but she is so loving that she just brushed it off. Audrey, my youngest (at this time), was just along for the ride in her carrier. I had a late night talk over a misunderstanding with my friend. I didn't get to bed until 12:00 am and I have a busy day for tomorrow. I worked out at home, but it was in between interruptions.

Today I ate:

Breakfast
All Bran cereal - ¾ cup with 1/3 cup 2% milk
Supplements: Multi-vitamin, EFA (essential fatty acids), and B-100
Drinks: green tea with Xylitol, and 16.9 oz of water

Lunch
5 almonds
Black - beans½ cup
1 drumstick
20 oz water

Dinner

10 almonds

TGIF spicy wings (didn't finish the serving, unfortunately they were fried & battered).

20 oz water

Evening Snack

16.9 oz water

For Fitness

Cardio - 20 minutes on the treadmill

Upper - 45 knee push-ups

It's Your Turn...

Day 9-_____

Journal Entry

_____

_____

_____

_____

_____

_____

_____

_____

_____

_____

_____

_____

_____

_____

_____

_____

Today I ate:

Breakfast

_____

_____

_____

_____

_____

_____

_____

_____

_____

Lunch

_____

_____

_____

_____

_____

_____

_____

_____

Dinner

_____

_____

_____

_____

_____

_____

_____

_____

Snack (max 2 a day)

_____

_____

_____

_____

For Fitness

Cardio -

_____

_____

Strength -

_____

_____

_____

_____

_____

Abs -

_____

_____

Day 10 – Wednesday, July 18th

Busy, busy, busy. Wow, I left the house late and I had a 9:30 appointment. I was rushing from one location to the next all day. I did get to make dinner and browse through several emails, but my workout was again pushed to the afternoon. This is good though; this means if you have a job and kids, you can still get a workout in before the day ends. My lunch was not well planned or executed.

Today I ate:

Breakfast
All Bran cereal - ¾ cup with 1/3 cup 2% milk
Supplements: Multi-vitamin, EFA (essential fatty acids), and B-100
Drinks: green tea with Xylitol, and 16.9 oz of water

Lunch
2 chicken tenders from Sonic
10 cashews
5 crackers with hummus
20 oz water

Dinner
Chicken sausage
Spinach
20 oz water

Evening Snack
16.9 oz water

For Fitness
Cardio - 35 minutes on the elliptical
Lower – Strength - 3 sets of 12 -machine leg press (110lb), 3 sets of 12 inner thigh and outer thigh gym machine (abductor/abduction), and 3 sets of 12 calve raises.
Abs -10 minutes of crunches and bicycles.

It's Your Turn…

Day 10-_____

Journal Entry

_____
_____
_____
_____
_____
_____
_____
_____
_____
_____
_____

Today I ate:

Breakfast

_____
_____
_____
_____
_____
_____
_____
_____

Lunch

_____
_____
_____
_____
_____

_____
_____
_____

Dinner

_____
_____
_____
_____
_____
_____
_____

Snack (max 2 a day)

_____
_____
_____

For Fitness
Cardio -

_____

Strength -

_____
_____
_____
_____

Abs -

_____

Day 11 – Thursday, July 19th

Today started out busy as usual, although it was very exciting. Tori and I had our first set of swim lessons. Wow, what a workout! Today was a good day. I did, however, eat a not-so-good diet today. A work in progress, yes!
Today I ate:

Breakfast
All Bran cereal - ¾ cup with 1/3 cup 2% milk
Supplements: Multi-vitamin, EFA (essential fatty acids), and B-100
Drinks: green tea with Xylitol, and 16.9 oz of water

Lunch
Half spicy chicken wrap - Chick-Fil-A
20 oz water

Dinner
Cauliflower - 1 cup
Spinach -1 cup
5 spicy wings
20 oz water

Evening Snack
16.9 oz water
10 animal crackers

For Fitness
Cardio - 45 minutes swim lessons.
Upper - 50 push-ups
50

Abs - 10 minutes of crunches and bicycles.

It's Your Turn...

Day 11-_____

Journal Entry

_____
_____
_____
_____
_____
_____
_____
_____
_____
_____
_____
_____
_____

Today I ate:

Breakfast

_____
_____
_____
_____
_____
_____
_____

Lunch

_____
_____
_____
_____
_____
_____
_____
_____
_____

Dinner

_____
_____
_____
_____
_____
_____
_____
_____

Snack (max 2 a day)

_____
_____
_____

For Fitness
Cardio -

_____

Strength -

_____

_____

_____

_____

_____

Abs -

_____

_____

Day 12 – Friday, July 20th

Today is home maintenance. I started my morning by working out in the house. I got the downstairs squared away, but I had to help my mom handle some business and then run errands, so I'll have to get to the upstairs later. I did get the girls bathroom done though! I am slowly transforming my eating, but next week I must push myself to the next level. It's time to transform my thinking about food. Today was a good day.

Today I ate:

Breakfast
All Bran cereal - ¾ cup with 1/3 cup 2% milk
Supplements: Multi-vitamin, EFA (essential fatty acids), and B-100
Drinks: green tea with Xylitol, and 16.9 oz of water

Lunch
Whole wheat pasta - 1 cup with chicken sausage
10 animal crackers
20 oz water

Dinner
Spinach -1 cup
3 hot wings
20 animal cookies
20 oz water

Evening Snack
16.9 oz water

For Fitness
Cardio - 30 minutes

It's Your Turn...

Day 12-_____

Journal Entry

_____
_____
_____
_____
_____
_____
_____
_____
_____
_____
_____
_____
_____
_____
_____

Today I ate:

Breakfast

_____

_____

_____

_____

_____

_____

_____

_____

Lunch

_____

_____

_____

_____

_____

_____

_____

Dinner

_____

_____

_____

_____

_____

_____

_____

Snack (max 2 a day)

_____

_____

_____

_____

For Fitness
Cardio -

_____

_____

Strength -

_____

_____

_____

_____

_____

Abs -

_____

_____

Day 13 – Saturday, July 21st

Today started off lovely. I was able to work out in the morning (at home) without any distractions. We had a birthday party to attend on the other side of town. I had to make sure I didn't have any pizza or cake. We had fun, and no cake or pizza... YAH! I did have some chicken wings from a local chicken joint...

Today I ate:

Breakfast

All Bran cereal - ¾ cup with 1/3 cup 2% milk
Supplements: Multi-vitamin, EFA (essential fatty acids), and B-100
Drinks: green tea with Xylitol, and 16.9 oz of water

Lunch
Salad

Dinner
8 wings
Green beans1 cup
20 oz water

Evening Snack
16.9 oz water

For Fitness
Cardio - 20 minutes
Upper/Strength - 3 sets of 12 -bicep curls, lateral raises, upright rows, triceps kickbacks, overhead triceps work, bicep curls again, and 15 (knee) pushups.
Abs

It's Your Turn...

Day 13-_____

Journal Entry

_____
_____
_____
_____
_____

_____
_____
_____
_____
_____
_____
_____
_____

Today I ate:

Breakfast

_____
_____
_____
_____
_____
_____
_____
_____

Lunch

_____
_____
_____
_____
_____
_____
_____
_____

Dinner

_____

_____

_____

_____

_____

_____

_____

_____

Snack (max 2 a day)

_____

_____

_____

For Fitness
Cardio -

_____

_____

Strength -

_____

_____

_____

_____

_____

Abs -

_____

_____

Day 14 – Sunday, July 22nd

Today was my scheduled "cheat day". However, I didn't have any dessert as I had planned. Some old friends stopped by so I made a nice home-cooked meal. We were busy in the house and I was on the phone for a while... it's always great to catch up with family. I can't believe Monday is almost here, but I am glad that I had the ability to navigate to another day.

Today I ate:

Breakfast
All Bran cereal - ¾ cup with 1/3 cup 2% milk
Supplements: Multi-vitamin, EFA (essential fatty acids), and B-100
Drinks: green tea with Xylitol, and 16.9 oz of water

Lunch
Spinach - 1 cup
1 chicken sausage
20 oz water

Dinner
Kidney beans - ½ cup
Brown rice - ½ cup
2-BBQ drumsticks
Cornbread (palm of my hand size slice)
Green beans - 1 cup
20 oz water

Evening Snack
16.9 oz water

For Fitness
None

It's Your Turn...

Day 14-_____

Journal Entry

_____
_____
_____
_____
_____
_____
_____
_____
_____
_____
_____
_____
_____
_____

Today I ate:

Breakfast

_____
_____
_____
_____
_____
_____
_____
_____

Lunch

_____
_____
_____
_____
_____
_____
_____
_____

Dinner

_____
_____
_____
_____
_____
_____
_____
_____

Snack (max 2 a day)

_____
_____
_____

For Fitness
Cardio -

_____

Strength -

_____

_____
_____
_____
_____
_____

Abs -

_____
_____

Day 15 – Monday, July 23rd

I joined a new brokerage today. The broker is really cool. I handled all my paperwork so I am official. We were so busy today. Kimmi didn't make it to camp because we couldn't find her pool shoes. I am attending a friend's "diaper shower" tonight, so that should be really fun. Talk with you tomorrow.

Today I ate:

Breakfast
Meal replacement shake
Supplements: Multi-vitamin, EFA (essential fatty acids), and B-100
20 oz water

Lunch
Chicken wrap
20 oz water

Dinner
Cilantro shrimp
Sautéed spinach
Salad
32 oz water

Evening Snack
16.9 oz water

For Fitness
Cardio - 30 minutes

It's Your Turn...

Day 15-_____

Journal Entry

_____
_____
_____
_____
_____
_____
_____
_____
_____
_____
_____
_____
_____
_____

Today I ate:

Breakfast

_____
_____
_____

_____
_____
_____
_____
_____
_____

Lunch

_____
_____
_____
_____
_____
_____
_____
_____

Dinner

_____
_____
_____
_____
_____
_____
_____
_____

Snack (max 2 a day)

_____
_____
_____
_____

For Fitness
Cardio -

_____

_____

Strength -

_____

_____

_____

_____

_____

Abs -

_____

_____

Day 16 – Tuesday, July 24th

I had my first meeting today with my new brokerage. The ladies I met were very friendly and spunky. I think this is going to be a great fit. I ran my oldest daughter to the doctors to check on her neck (muscle spasm from swimming lessons). She is doing better, and we will administer Ibuprofen for a day or so. I was then swamped with dinner duties and so forth. I skipped my workout and ate with less control, which kind of sucks, but I will not be defeated!

Today I ate:

Breakfast
Meal replacement shake
Supplements: Multi-vitamin, EFA (essential fatty acids), and B-100
20 oz water

Lunch
Chicken salad
20 oz water

Dinner
Salmon
32 oz water

Evening Snack
5 wings
10 oz water

For Fitness
None - I know - what I am doing, right?

It's Your Turn...

Day 16.9-_____

Journal Entry

_____

_____

_____

_____

_____

_____

_____

_____

_____

_____

_____

Today I ate:

Breakfast

_____

_____

_____

_____

_____

_____

_____

_____

Lunch

_____

_____

_____

_____

_____

_____

_____

_____

Dinner

_____

_____

_____

_____

_____

_____
_____
_____

Snack (max 2 a day)

_____
_____
_____
_____

For Fitness
Cardio -

_____
_____

Strength -

_____
_____
_____
_____
_____
_____

Abs -

_____
_____

Day 17 – Wednesday, July 25th

Today was pretty good. I got a workout in during the morning hours, and a few more minutes in the afternoon. I'm stoked. I got several things knocked off my "To Do List", and was able to work on some things that I enjoy in the later part of the evening.

Today I ate:

Breakfast
Meal replacement shake
Supplements: Multi-vitamin, EFA (essential fatty acids), and B-100
20 oz water

Lunch
Salmon & salad (lettuce & chunky spicy salsa)
20 oz water

Dinner
Spinach -1 cup
Chicken apple sausage link -1
Small sliver of cornbread -1
32 oz water

Evening Snack
Salad
10 oz water

For Fitness
Cardio - 35 minutes of cardio
Upper/Strength - 3 sets of 12 – bicep curls, lateral raises, upright rows, triceps kickbacks, overhead triceps work, bicep curls again, and 25 (knee) pushups. 2 sets of 12 - biceps curls, lateral raises, and triceps kickbacks.

It's Your Turn...

Day 17-_____

Journal Entry

_____

_____

_____

_____

_____

_____

_____

_____

_____

_____

_____

_____

Today I ate:

Breakfast

_____

_____

_____

_____

_____

_____

_____

_____

Lunch

_____

_____

_____

_____
_____
_____
_____
_____

Dinner

_____
_____
_____
_____
_____
_____
_____

Snack (max 2 a day)

_____
_____
_____

For Fitness
Cardio -

_____

Strength -

_____
_____
_____
_____
_____

Abs -

_____

_____

Day 18 – Thursday, July 26th

Oh my goodness, today was so busy! I had to maneuver time between working out, swimming lessons for Tori, and a doctor appointment for me. I got some type of bacteria in my eye. I was busy all day doing one thing or the other, and laundry never ends...

Today I ate:

Breakfast
Meal replacement shake
Supplements: Multi-vitamin, EFA (essential fatty acids), and B-100
20 oz water

Lunch
Brown rice ½ cup
Chicken sausage ½ link
Spinach - ½ cup

Dinner
Spinach -½ cup
Chicken breast (grilled)
Mashed potatoes - 3 tablespoons
1 large piece of cornbread
32 oz water

Evening Snack

10 oz water

For Fitness

Cardio - 30 minutes of cardio
Lower - 3 sets of abduction, adduction, and calf raises

It's Your Turn...

Day 18-_____

Journal Entry

_____
_____
_____
_____
_____
_____
_____
_____
_____
_____
_____
_____
_____
_____

Today I ate:

Breakfast

_____
_____
_____
_____

_____
_____
_____
_____
_____

Lunch

_____
_____
_____
_____
_____
_____
_____
_____

Dinner

_____
_____
_____
_____
_____
_____
_____
_____

Snack (max 2 a day)

_____
_____
_____
_____

For Fitness
Cardio -

_____

_____

Strength -

_____

_____

_____

_____

_____

Abs -

_____

_____

Day 19 – Friday, July 27th

   Today was fantastic. I got an awesome report from the doctor. No thyroid problems. I got my vehicle signage changed over to my new company, and it looks great. We had lunch as a family. Kimmi got her cochlear fixed and received her replacement back up. The kids and I went shopping at Michael's for some crafts, and then they had California Pizza Kitchen, and I didn't even flinch. We watched a family movie: Left Behind. Today was super.
   Today I ate:

Breakfast
Meal replacement shake
Supplements: Multi-vitamin, EFA (essential fatty acids), and B-100
20 oz water

Lunch
Chicken wrap
20 oz water

Dinner
Salad with spicy salsa
Chicken breast (grilled)
20 oz water

Evening Snack
10 oz water
½ bag Newman's popcorn

For Fitness
Cardio - 20 minutes of circuit cardio
Upper - 3 sets of 12 - bicep curls, lateral raises, upright rows, triceps kickbacks, overhead triceps work, bicep curls again, and 25 (knee) pushups
Abs

It's Your Turn...

Day 19-_____

Journal Entry
_____
_____
_____
_____
_____
_____
_____
_____

_____

_____

_____

_____

_____

_____

Today I ate:

Breakfast

_____

_____

_____

_____

_____

_____

_____

_____

Lunch

_____

_____

_____

_____

_____

_____

_____

_____

Dinner

_____

_____

_____
_____
_____
_____
_____
_____
_____

Snack (max 2 a day)

_____
_____
_____
_____

For Fitness

Cardio -

_____
_____

Strength -

_____
_____
_____
_____
_____

Abs -

_____
_____

Day 20 - Saturday, July 28th

Today was another awesome day. We didn't leave the house. It was nice to just relax and get extra organizing done.

I felt really good today. I needed the rest.
Today I ate:

Breakfast
Meal replacement shake
Supplements: Multi-vitamin, EFA (essential fatty acids), and B-100
20 oz water

Lunch
Chicken breast with spicy salsa
Lettuce and tomato with 1 tablespoon olive oil

Dinner
Salad with spicy salsa
Chicken breast (grilled)
20 oz water

Evening Snack
10 oz water
½ bag Newman's popcorn

For Fitness
Cardio - 30 minutes of circuit cardio
Abs

It's Your Turn...

Day 20-_____

Journal Entry

_____

_____

_____
_____
_____
_____
_____
_____
_____
_____
_____
_____

Today I ate:

<u>Breakfast</u>

_____
_____
_____
_____
_____
_____
_____
_____

<u>Lunch</u>

_____
_____
_____
_____
_____
_____

_____

_____

Dinner

_____

_____

_____

_____

_____

_____

_____

_____

Snack (max 2 a day)

_____

_____

_____

For Fitness
Cardio -

_____

Strength -

_____

_____

_____

_____

Abs -

_____

Day 21 – Sunday, July 29th

I went to bed at a reasonably decent hour last night, so I feel refreshed. Today was my "cheat day". Every Sunday is my "cheat day". I am working up the will power not be a totally insane eater on this day. I am actually proud of myself. I would usually eat a whole bag of chips from Qdoba, along with an ice-cream treat from one of the creamery shops. Not this week. Feeling good...go Mom, it's your birthday!

Today I ate:

Breakfast
Tuna kit - no mayo, sweet relish and 5 crackers
Supplements: Multi-vitamin, EFA (essential fatty acids), and B-100
20 oz water

Lunch
Chicken and beef nachos from Qdoba (only 5 chips) - made with beans, lettuce, pico, cheese, and spicy salsa
20 oz water

Dinner
½ California Pizza Kitchen (mini) -Jamaican Jerk Chicken Salad with Italian
20 oz water

Evening Snack

For Fitness
Cardio -1 hour cycling at YMCA
Abs

It's Your Turn...

Day 21-_____

Journal Entry

_____
_____
_____
_____
_____
_____
_____
_____
_____
_____
_____
_____
_____

Today I ate:

Breakfast

_____
_____
_____
_____
_____
_____
_____
_____

Lunch

_____
_____
_____
_____
_____
_____
_____
_____

Dinner

_____
_____
_____
_____
_____
_____
_____

Snack (max 2 a day)

_____
_____
_____

For Fitness
Cardio -

_____
_____

Strength -

_____

_____

_____

_____

_____

_____

Abs -

_____

_____

Day 22 – Monday, July 30th

I woke up again refreshed. We didn't have anywhere to be today, and that was nice. I wasn't able to work out in the morning due to a few unforeseen tasks, but I got it in this afternoon. It was killer circuit cardio... my legs are humming! Today was a good day.

Today I ate:

Breakfast
Tuna kit - no mayo, sweet relish and 5 crackers.
Supplements: Multi-vitamin, EFA (essential fatty acids), and B-100
20 oz water

Lunch
Chicken salad with Italian dressing.
20 oz water

Dinner
Lentils ½ cup
Green beans 2/3 cup
Palm size chicken breast.

Evening Snack
15 pretzels

For Fitness
Cardio - 35 minutes of circuit cardio
Upper - DVD (Firm Parts), 45 push-ups
Abs

It's Your Turn...

Day 22-_____

Journal Entry

_____

_____

_____

_____

_____

_____

_____

_____

_____

_____

_____

_____

_____

Today I ate:

Breakfast

_____
_____
_____
_____
_____
_____
_____
_____

Lunch

_____
_____
_____
_____
_____
_____
_____
_____

Dinner

_____
_____
_____
_____
_____
_____
_____
_____

Snack (max 2 a day)

_____
_____

_____

_____

For Fitness
Cardio -

_____

Strength -

_____

_____

_____

_____

_____

Abs -

_____

_____

Day 23 – Tuesday, July 31st

Today was rather busy. I met with my broker at around 11 and I received my first live lead and will be traveling all over Middle TN to find them a home. The family is relocating. I'm very excited, and hope to serve them well. I worked out in the morning. My evening was swamped. This is so exciting.

Today I ate:

Breakfast
Tuna kit - no mayo, sweet relish and 5 crackers.
Supplements: Multi-vitamin, EFA (essential fatty acids), and B-100
20 oz water

Lunch
Chicken salad with Italian dressing.
20 oz water

Dinner
Lentils ½ cup
Green beans 2/3 cup
Palm size chicken breast

Evening Snack

For Fitness
Cardio - 35 minutes of circuit cardio
Abs

It's Your Turn…

Day 23-_____

Journal Entry

_____
_____
_____
_____
_____
_____
_____
_____
_____
_____
_____
_____

Today I ate:

Breakfast

_____
_____
_____
_____
_____
_____
_____

Lunch

_____
_____
_____
_____
_____
_____
_____

Dinner

_____
_____
_____
_____
_____

_____

_____

Snack (max 2 a day)

_____

_____

_____

_____

For Fitness
Cardio -

_____

_____

Strength -

_____

_____

_____

_____

_____

Abs -

_____

_____

Day 24 – Wednesday, Aug 1st

Wow. Today was busy. I spent most of my day in a new town about an hour and half away from my area. My clients really like one of the homes we viewed. I didn't work out today and I really feel bad about it, but I had to get all those directions together and fax maps to my client. We are going to a totally different area tomorrow. I should have worked out first thing in the morning. My dinner was fried chicken. I know,

what I am doing is not right, but at least it was white meat...
yeah that makes it better.

Today I ate:

Breakfast
Tuna kit - no mayo, sweet relish and 5 crackers.
Supplements: Multi-vitamin, EFA (essential fatty acids), and B-100
20 oz water

Lunch
Chicken salad with Italian dressing.
20 oz water

Dinner
2 pieces Popeye's chicken.
30 oz water

Evening Snack

For Fitness
None

It's Your Turn...

Day 24-_____

Journal Entry

_____
_____
_____
_____
_____

_____
_____
_____
_____
_____
_____
_____
_____
_____

Today I ate:

<u>Breakfast</u>

_____
_____
_____
_____
_____
_____
_____
_____
_____

<u>Lunch</u>

_____
_____
_____
_____
_____
_____
_____
_____
_____

Dinner

_____
_____
_____
_____
_____
_____
_____
_____
_____

Snack (max 2 a day)

_____
_____
_____
_____

For Fitness

Cardio -

_____
_____

Strength -

_____
_____
_____
_____
_____

Abs -

_____
_____

Day 25 – Thursday, Aug 2nd

Today was a longer but better day in my mind, since I worked out in the morning. We visited a few homes, but none compared to the home in the area. We drove 2.5 hours in the other direction to view the home. It was long, but I wanted to ensure my clients were satisfied and felt extremely satisfied with their decision. Once we arrived, they fell back in love with it. Today was long, but what an experience. We are writing an offer tomorrow! Whoo Hoo!

Today I ate:

Breakfast
Tuna kit - no mayo, sweet relish and 5 crackers.
Supplements: Multi-vitamin, EFA (essential fatty acids), and B-100
20 oz water

Lunch
MRP bar
20 oz water

Dinner
Lentils ½ cup
Green beans 2/3 cup
Palm size chicken breast

Evening Snack
15 pretzels

For Fitness
Cardio - 35 minutes of circuit cardio
Upper - DVD (Firm Parts), 45 push-ups
Abs

It's Your Turn...

Day 25-_____

Journal Entry

_____
_____
_____
_____
_____
_____
_____
_____
_____
_____
_____
_____

Today I ate:

Breakfast

_____
_____
_____
_____
_____
_____
_____
_____

Lunch

_____
_____
_____
_____
_____
_____
_____
_____
_____

Dinner

_____
_____
_____
_____
_____
_____
_____
_____

Snack (max 2 a day)

_____
_____
_____

For Fitness
Cardio -

_____
_____

Strength -

_____

_____

_____

_____

_____

_____

Abs -

_____

_____

Day 26 – Friday, Aug 3rd

Wow, from the jump I was running. The lights went out so I woke up an hour late. No time to work out this morning. I had to get the kids to day care and then get to my office to get my documents together. Everything went off without a hitch (well a few extra questions on my part). I sent the contract and got a verbal yes by the end of the day. WOW! This is so exciting. I got my workout in during the afternoon, and got some shopping done for the kids. I smoked it today, baby…

Today I ate:

Breakfast
Tuna kit - no mayo, sweet relish and 5 crackers.
Supplements: Multi-vitamin, EFA (essential fatty acids), and B-100
20 oz water

Lunch
Chicken salad with Italian dressing.
20 oz water

Dinner
Lentils ½ cup

Green beans 2/3 cup
Palm size chicken breast

Evening Snack
15 pretzels

For Fitness
Cardio - 35 minutes of circuit cardio
Lower - 3 sets of squats, abduction, adduction, and calf raises.
Abs

It's Your Turn...

Day 26-_____

Journal Entry

_____
_____
_____
_____
_____
_____
_____
_____
_____
_____
_____
_____
_____
_____

Today I ate:

Breakfast

_____
_____
_____
_____
_____
_____
_____
_____

Lunch

_____
_____
_____
_____
_____
_____
_____
_____

Dinner

_____
_____
_____
_____
_____
_____
_____

Snack (max 2 a day)

_____
_____
_____
_____

For Fitness
Cardio -

_____
_____

Strength -

_____
_____
_____
_____
_____
_____

Abs -

_____
_____

Day 27 – Saturday, Aug 4th

Today was early and busy. It is tax-free weekend so we had to get out and get the savings while we could…you can understand my sense of urgency with four girls. Wow, the day was really long, but we got the major stuff done. Tomorrow is our first Sunday family meal. I am starting a tradition. Every first Sunday is family dinner. Moreover, it's my cheat day.

Today I ate:

Breakfast
Meal replacement shake.
Supplements: Multi-vitamin, EFA (essential fatty acids), and B-102

100
20 oz water

Lunch
Chicken nuggets.

Dinner
Chicken
Brown rice

Evening Snack

For Fitness
Walked the mall (Tax-free weekend) with 4 children/2 strollers

It's Your Turn...

Day 27-_____

Journal Entry

_____
_____
_____
_____
_____
_____
_____
_____
_____
_____
_____
_____
_____

Today I ate:

Breakfast

_____
_____
_____
_____
_____
_____
_____
_____
_____

Lunch

_____
_____
_____
_____
_____
_____
_____
_____
_____

Dinner

_____
_____
_____
_____
_____
_____

_____

_____

Snack (max 2 a day)

_____

_____

_____

_____

For Fitness
Cardio -

_____

_____

Strength -

_____

_____

_____

_____

_____

Abs -

_____

_____

Day 28 – Sunday, Aug 5th

Today flew by. After church, I had to get to cooking, and I cooked till 5:00 pm. It was our first family meal (Mom & Uncle). I plan to expand it to friends but that can get expensive. I ate more than I planned (2 slices), but it's my cheat day.
Today I ate:

Breakfast
All Bran
Supplements: Multi-vitamin, EFA (essential fatty acids), and B-100
20 oz water

Lunch
Thin slice oven California Pizza Kitchen
20 oz water

Dinner
Pork chop (½ piece)
Mac 'N Cheese (2/3 cup)
Salad
Corn (1 ear)
Chocolate chip pound cake (2 slices)
20 oz water

Evening Snack

For Fitness
None

It's Your Turn...

Day 28-_____

Journal Entry
_____
_____
_____
_____
_____

Today I ate:

Breakfast

Lunch

Dinner

_____
_____
_____
_____
_____
_____
_____
_____
_____
_____

Snack (max 2 a day)

_____
_____
_____
_____

For Fitness
Cardio -

_____
_____

Strength -

_____
_____
_____
_____
_____
_____

Abs -

_____
_____

Day 29 – Monday, Aug 6th

Today was an awesome day. I got to sleep in until 8:00... that is late for me. I made it to the Y for a workout class, and I got lots of work done. I am going to have to reschedule some things in my life in order to maintain balance in the areas that are important. I have an office meeting tomorrow so I had better get some rest.

Today I ate:

Breakfast
Lentils ½ cup
Supplements: Multi-vitamin, EFA (essential fatty acids), and B-100
20 oz water

Lunch
1 deviled egg
Salad (soy ginger dressing, 2 tablespoons, lettuce, tomato, onion, few croutons)
20 oz water

Dinner
Pork chop (½ piece)
Green salad
20 oz water

Evening Snack
Jalapeño almonds (handful)

For Fitness
1 hour Zumba (aerobics Latin dance/exercise)
10 minutes on elliptical
Upper - 3 set of biceps & triceps kickbacks (left shoulder hurts - I'm taking it easy)

Abs

It's Your Turn...

Day 29-_____

Journal Entry

_____
_____
_____
_____
_____
_____
_____
_____
_____
_____
_____
_____
_____

Today I ate:

Breakfast

_____
_____
_____
_____
_____
_____
_____

Lunch

Dinner

Snack (max 2 a day)

For Fitness
Cardio -

Strength -

_____

_____

_____

_____

_____

_____

Abs -

_____

_____

Day 30 – Tuesday, Aug 7th

Well, today is the big day. Thirty days of journaling, body and mind training. I'm excited. I can now transition into some hard core training (after I get my shoulder checked out). My next journaling pattern may be much more goal-oriented. Talk with you soon.
Today I ate:

Breakfast
All Bran
Supplements: Multi-vitamin, EFA (essential fatty acids), and B-100
20 oz water

Lunch
Chicken salad
20 oz water

Dinner
Chicken breast
Lentils ½ cup

Salad
20 oz water

Evening Snack
GNU Bar

For Fitness
30 minutes of circuit cardio

It's Your Turn...

Day 30-_____

Journal Entry

_____
_____
_____
_____
_____
_____
_____
_____
_____
_____
_____
_____
_____
_____

Today I ate:

Breakfast

_____

_____

_____

_____

_____

_____

_____

_____

Lunch

_____

_____

_____

_____

_____

_____

_____

_____

Dinner

_____

_____

_____

_____

_____

_____

_____

Snack (max 2 a day)

_____

_____

For Fitness

Cardio -

Strength -

Abs -

Congratulations...If you are reading this, success is yours. You have toiled the pressure, urges, and crossed the finish line as a winner against the race for good health.

Room 2
BOOT CAMP BODY

Hello, and welcome to some hard-core training. If you have recently finished room 1 and are about to step it up, I congratulate and applaud your entry. If you are visiting this room already in "contest" mode I welcome you as well.

Let's get down to the nitty gritty.

What I've applied in this section is all my military training. Let's face it, there is no magic pill, and the there's no magic drink. You shouldn't want to look like anyone else but you. You are the celebrity, you are an original. So be the best YOU that you can be. Stay with me now…

This is a very simple but highly effective approach to getting that phenomenal body that you desire. You won't be hungry, you don't have to join a gym, and you don't need a calculator or booklet for this plan. All you need is the will power and the motivation. I know you have both of these within you, or you wouldn't be reading this book right now.

I'm going to give you what you want up front. I don't want to bore you with tons of facts, figures, and finds. I do have some extended health building tips, but they are in the rears (another room in the book).

I want you to feel marvelous, look phenomenal, and maintain this health, long-term so that you can focus on your purpose in life with freedom from weight and health concerns.

You can visit my website at www.bloggersdiet.com for awesome tools that will assist you in the mission of pulling out the fit & fabulous you.

Change is inevitable in this life; will your change be towards a healthier, fitter and happier you? You decide.

A moment to reflect

The way you see yourself today will affect your performance today. Zig Ziglar

For we live by believing, not by seeing. 2 Corinthians 5:7 (NLT)

I'll be using lots of military jargon along the way but don't worry, I'll explain myself at all times. I'm your personal Drill Sergeant and I will be pushing you to excellence. Check out my website for extra motivation at www.bloggersdiet.com.

It's all really simple, here are the battles:
  - The battle to fight the food addiction,
  - The battle to fight poor eating habits,
  - The battle to change tradition,
  - The battle of the mind,
  - The battle to stay committed to good health.

I am with you, and you ARE ready... Let's win the war!

Make no mistake; you will have to put forth maximum effort. Days will come when you will want to give up, when you want to fall out and resort back to your undisciplined ways, but if you push forward, down the path less traveled, you will achieve maximum results. You will accomplish goals that you set yourself years ago, and conquer new ones.

You have passed the entrance exam. Before I got my foot in the door to serving my country, I had to take an aptitude test for the privilege of joining the U.S. Army. You have already passed! If you are still reading at this point, you are ready. All

I need from you now is for you to sign your Enlistment Documents. Once I decided I was going to make my move from civilian to soldier, I was required to sign various commitment letters, one of which is known as an Enlistment Document. The form basically stated that I would commit to the U.S. Army for a certain period of time. Below, you will find your commitment letter. You are committing to me that you are going to make this a lifetime change, and that you are going to work diligently towards achieving success, but most of all, you're signing up for a new YOU.

You can burn a copy (print a copy) of this, or visit my website and print a copy.

Enlistment Letter

I, _____, agree to begin my training on this day, _____,

- ➤ I agree to put forth all my efforts into attaining tons of energy, a healthy mind, and a totally fit body.
- ➤ I will make every effort to be tightened, toned, and terrific.
- ➤ I will not allow food to run me; I will control it because I am in charge.
- ➤ I realize that my body is a wonderfully made temple that I must maintain with high regard and high standards.
- ➤ I will not allow non health-conscious individuals to discourage me. I deserve to be and feel my best at all times.
- ➤ I choose NOW to leave laziness and excessive food consumption behind.
- ➤ I am creating a new way that will keep me healthy for years to come.
- ➤ I have told _____ about my journey because they are a part of my support system, and they agree to encourage me to drive forward.

Nothing can stop me now except myself, and I have the ability to control and change me.

Signature_____
Date_____

Post this in an area where you will see it daily as a reminder of your commitment.

Area 1
THE SHAKE DOWN

After I had signed my paperwork, got my bags all packed, gave hugs to family; I was bussed along with other recruits to the training camp that would become home for the next few weeks. Upon arrival, several Drill Sergeants awaited us in the wee hours of the morning. They were ready to prepare us for the long journey ahead. After being hustled off the bus with shouting and wailing from the Drill Sergeants, we had what is known as a shake down. Basically, you dump all your baggage and you get rid of anything that isn't essential to your transformation.

So guess what...

It's SHAKE DOWN time.

I told you in the introduction that I would make it simple and easy, so here we go. The list below contains all the things you need to rid your house of.

FOODS THAT ROB YOU OF GOOD HEALTH & ENERGY 'THE KILLER LIST'
Anything containing high fructose corn syrup
Artificial colors
Artificial sweeteners: aspartame, saccharin, sucralose, acesfulfame-K
Bacon & sausage
Candy
Canned fruit

Canned vegetables
Doughnuts
Foods that contain Trans fats (read the ingredients labels and look for partially hydrogenated oils)
High sugar cereals
Luncheon meats that are less than 95% fat free, or contain sodium nitrates
Margarine & lard
Non-dairy creamers
Snack chips
Sodas (regular or diet)
Sodium nitrate
White flour products

Area 2
BASE CONTROL

What is a base? A base has many definitions. Here are a few: the foundation, the support unit, a place from where you draw supplies, the fundamental groundwork and the main ingredient.

Your base is your kitchen, pantry, and cabinets.

You want to consume lots of fruits, vegetables, whole grains, legumes, and lean proteins. You want to significantly decrease, with the intention to eliminate, packaged cupcakes, doughnuts, white flour, white sugar, high fat/high salt chips, sodas, and candy.

What I don't want you to do is starve yourself. You need to eat at least three meals a day, with two snacks between meals. I know this sounds strange, but trust me, it works. Remember, we're changing the kinds of foods we eat and the portions we consume, which will yield superb results. Let's make portion control simple. Any meats should be no bigger than the palm of your hand. Any brown rice or whole wheat pasta should be a tennis ball portion or use an ice-cream scooper to serve it. Vegetables you can have in abundance.

As I mentioned earlier, you should eat three meals a day with two snacks along the way, so if you are skipping breakfast and your goal is to lose weight, you are reversing the weight loss process. Not eating breakfast puts your body into starvation mode, which means that your body begins to store (hold onto) fat in order to function properly.

Skipping breakfast not only sends your body into starvation mode, but it also slows down your metabolism. You rob yourself of the energy that is needed to start your mornings strong, and skipping breakfast promotes foggy thinking. You will also find yourself famished before it is time for lunch. I don't want you running down to the snack machine for a soda and a candy bar. The carbs (simple carbohydrates) from those items will give you a momentary sugar spike. This spike is short-lived. When your blood sugar begins to level out, it sinks a little lower than normal and you will be sluggish and hungry all over again.

Area 3
BASIC TRAINING... ONLY THE STRONG SURVIVE!

Now that you have the fundamentals, it's time to get started into a rigorous re-training that is going to rock your world.

My basic training was actually 8 weeks of training and self-realization. Your basic training phase is 14 to 28 days, depending on what you decide after day 14. I call this period operation Clean Sweep. You are reversing the way your mind thinks about food, and forcing the body into submission during this period.

First, here are your allowed foods during this period:

SEAFOOD
All fish

POULTRY
Turkey breast
Chicken breast-skinless/boneless

NUTS/FATS/CHEESE/EGGS/SEASONINGS
Cashews, walnuts, flax, hazelnut, macadamia
Raw almonds
Eggs (more whites)
Olive oil
Dijon mustard
Regular mustard
Seasoning blends that don't add sugar & salt
Red wine vinegar

VEGATABLES
All but limit corn and no white potatoes; the greener the vegetable... the better!

LEGUMES
Lentils
Black beans

Chick peas
FRUIT
All berries
Green apple
Lemon and lime
BEVERAGES AND MISCELLANOUS
WATER
Green tea
Black tea
Multi-vitamin
CLA (check your local health food store)
Protein shake-mix with water (twice a day: pre-workout with a fruit, and post workout without fruit)
Your personally selected fat burner (Ripped Fuel, Cytolean, Lipo-6 or the like)
EFA (Essential Fatty Acids)
Oatmeal (not instant) or high protein cereal
Brown rice
Broths - low sodium

I know it may seem drastic, but drastic will give you results. Really, it's not drastic, it's simply about changing the way you view food. Food isn't a celebration commodity, a pleasure giver, or a time passing object; its only goal is to provide nutrition to help you sustain life. These foods will provide you with good living. Along with this, remember not to eat anything two hours prior to bedtime. This allows your body time to rejuvenate, rest, and restore, instead of working all night to digest food. You can prepare your meals in any fashion, as long as you choose from this list only. Each meal must contain one portion of protein, carbohydrate, and fat. Your desserts are fruit and tea!

A popular quote states, "If you don't make time for your health, you'll have to make time for your illness." Think about it!

Here is a sample plan of how a day of eating should look:

Breakfast:
High protein cold cereal, non-fat milk with 2 eggs (boiled or scrambled) OR
Oatmeal (not instant) with 2 eggs

Snack (2-3 hours later):
Protein shake, protein bar, 15 nuts with 1 fruit, or 1 can tuna (no mayo).

Lunch:
4 oz protein, heaped serving of green vegetable, ½ cup brown rice, sweet potato, lentils, or black beans.

Snack (2-3 hours later):
Protein shake, protein bar, 15 nuts with 1 fruit, or 1 can tuna (no mayo).

Dinner:
4 oz protein, heaped serving of green vegetables, fruit of your choice.

You can mix foods from the approved list above, but stick to the basic guideline of portions and nutrients that I listed in the sample above to achieve your maximum results.

THE FREEBIE

Since this is a highly strict regimen that could last for up to one month, I have included a 'breakaway day'. On any given day per week, you can feel free to have something that would be considered a 'cheat food'. Let's say you decide to make this day on Sunday; you can feel free to have one meal or food item that is indulgent to the palate but not necessarily to the body. You do not *have* to use this day, it is optional! The idea behind the breakaway day is that you understand your limits, you exercise self-control, and you trick the brain into thinking not NO, but not NOW!

So, you have your allowed foods; let's give you the run down on your fitness regimen.

I want you to do 20 to 45 minutes of cardio five times a week (walking, jogging, swimming, elliptical, or jumping rope) in the morning. Fitness in the morning helps boost your brain function, and alerts your body to burn calories all day. If for whatever reason, you can't work out in the morning, try to get it in by lunchtime. I say by lunchtime because during this period, you will exercise again before dinner, another 20 to 30 minutes of cardio. The goal of your cardio sessions is to burn 150 to 200 calories in as least amount of time as possible. If you aren't working on a machine, then investing in a calorie counter might be useful.

In conjunction with your workout, you should do three days a week of muscle building training.

Exercise will give you the results you want to see sooner. Cardiovascular training will improve your general well-being, burn extra fat, and it will definitely boost your energy levels.

Doing some muscle toning workouts will also define the areas that we like to see in shape. Cardiovascular exercise improves the functioning of the heart and the lungs. Your cardio can come in the form of walking, jogging, stepping, or cycling, for at least 20 minutes.

If you can afford to join a gym or fitness club, this will be great! For those who can't, I have included great workouts that you can do in the privacy of your own home. These exercises will help to improve your muscle tone, boost your metabolism, accelerate fat loss, and help burn calories. You can always tweak the exercises to your level of comfort, but progressively increase intensity every two to three weeks. If possible, you can also purchase some awesome workout DVDs. I like Billy Blanks, Denise Austin, Jeanette Jenkins, Tamilee Web, Minna Lessig, and any of the 10-minute solutions series.

Getting a partner during this phase is also a great motivational tool. You can visit my website to blog your feelings, join an online group, or sign up to receive personalized plans and coaching specialized for you. In the military, we had what was called a battle buddy. Your battle buddy is and does just what the name states: goes to battle with you, knows where you are, and what's going on, and supports you in every way.

Another quote I love goes like this, "The definition of insanity is doing the same thing over and over, but expecting a different result." If you are going to do something repeatedly, then let it be something that is good for your health.

After your 14 to 28 days are over, you can personally access how you want to move forward. I recommend adding in more whole grain and fruit after 28 days for variety (more information in next area). Sticking to this eating plan will keep you feeling energized, looking young, and ready to conquer life.

128

Tip: Poor eating habits usually make people feel like they can't exercise. This is all the more reason to go work out.

Area 4
AIT (ADVANCED INDIVIDUAL TRAINING)

Now that you are armed with a new attitude on food and yourself, the real journey begins.

AIT is where new recruits go after they finish basic training. This is where I learned the skills that would become my military profession. This is where everything I learned in basic training would be built upon and challenged.

AIT for you should begin immediately after the basic training phase. If you believe that you have mastered the mind, and overcome your reliance on sugar and nutrition-less food, then you are ready.

The major changes in this phase are that you can add in whole grains and more fruit of your choice (see chart below).

GRAINS	FRUIT
100% Whole or sprouted grains	All fruit
RED MEAT	**FATS, OILS, NUTS, DAIRY**
Sirloin, remove the fat	Coconut butter & oil
Tenderloin, remove the fat	Natural peanut butter
	Yogurt
	Honey

ALWAYS STAY AWAY FROM FOODS LISTED IN 'THE KILLER LIST'

You are also monitoring your portion control by keeping a journal mentally or physically of roughly how many calories you are consuming per day.

This is simple: whatever weight you want to be, multiple it by 10 and that is about how many calories you should consume per day. So, let's say Angela wants to keep her weight at around 130 lbs, her daily caloric intake should be around 1300 calories give or take.

You are, at this point, fully aware that YOU are in control of your eating, so this is easy. Mind over matter!

If you are a person who enjoys keeping up with the numbers very closely in your diet, I have made it a little simpler for you. Below, you will find three nutrition content plans that you can implement during this phase.

The 1300-calorie plan is the first plan which can be used. The macronutrient breakdown I like to use is a 40/35/25 split.

Carbohydrates Per Day	Protein Per Day	Fat Per Day
130 grams carbs	113 grams (you can round up)	36 grams of fat
Neutral or less is fine	More is fine	Less is fine

These plans are based on you eating five meals per day. If you decide to have a breakfast that has 0 grams of fat, you can save those grams to be used on another meal, as long as you don't go over your combined limit. You can also ignore the fact that you have left over fat grams and continue on as normal, this creates a deficit that is good for your health, and great for your waistline!

The 1600-calorie plan is second. This would allow for 320 calories per meal. These plans are based on you eating five meals per day.

Carbohydrates Per Day	Protein Per Day	Fat Per Day
160	140	44

The next plan is the 1900 + calorie plan, which should be used by **competitive athletes, body builders, and individuals with high metabolism**. This would allow for 380 calories per meal.

Carbohydrates Per Day	Protein Per Day	Fat Per Day
190	166	52

As you can see, the plans are broken up in a way that allows each person to choose an area that suits their needs.

The 1300-calorie plan is used for weight loss.

The 1600-calorie plan is used for weight loss and weight management.

The 1900 calories plan is best for competitive athletes, body builders, and individuals with very high metabolisms.

You don't need to carry a calculator or tablet for journaling forever, but this will be helpful in the beginning to give yourself a visual understanding of what you are consuming. This is just a guideline, a tool to assist you in being conscious of what you are eating. You now have the freedom to take charge of your health. You can fuel your tank with foods that nourish it, and keep it running for miles, or you can fuel it with garbage that robs you of your destiny. The choice is always yours. I believe in you, but you have to believe in yourself! I did it and I know you can do it too!

Tip 1: You should constantly remind yourself that your current regimen will only keep you where you are at, and change will take you where you want to be.

Tip 2: Learning to change our habits should be done in balance, and in the right mindset. We are not looking to just lose a few pounds; we are looking to make total lifestyle changes that will equip us with healthy bodies, to keep us feeling and looking good for many days to come.

Area 5
PERMANENT DUTY - RESIDING IN THE NEW YOU!

If you have followed the steps laid out before you, at this point it is smooth sailing. Cravings are few, if any, and control is very prevalent in your life.

You should have realized at this point that calories in versus calories out will keep the excess weight off. The substances of your food with keep you healthy long-term.

Being fit means something different to every individual, and this is a good thing. There is a lot of media influence to look a certain way; tall, six-packed, big muscles for guys, skinny legs for ladies, no facial blemishes, and long hair. There is absolutely nothing wrong with any of those things. What is wrong is the representation of those things, and how this representation is shaping the minds of many Americans.

We are all uniquely and wonderfully made. Everyone is blessed with a spectacular look. It's your own look... an original is what you are. So let's not spend time or money into fitting some stereotype of what beautiful is. Let's think about this; they give you fast food, they tell you more is better, and you work so hard that you neglect body, mind, and soul.

Accept where you are, love who you are, realize that change is inevitable, and the type of change you experience is up to you. Instead of focusing on the symptoms, search deeper for the root of the problem. This may require counseling from a therapist, clergy, a pastor, or a really grounded friend. Once you can see the problem, make a plan to fix it.

Some things to incorporate into your life might include: uplifting music, prayer, Bible study, healthy fulfilling relationships, aromatherapy, and a good night's sleep! Invest in extra-curricular activities that feed your soul. We are who we are. It is our job as humans to take care of what we have to our best ability. Do things because you desire to do them for personal satisfaction, not to look, feel, or be like someone else. Do you!

To the goal-oriented, you could sit down with yourself, get a pen and paper then write, "What is fit to me and why?" Then I want you to answer your question, print it out, and keep it in a place where you can remind yourself of your own personal goal, not someone else's.

Please keep in mind that nothing happens over night, and anything worth having will not come easy. So please try to stay off the scales. I want you to chart your weight and body measurements the day before you begin your Boot Camp Body plan. You can keep track of this using my weight-tracking program, or you can create something on your own, as long as you can pinpoint your changes, that's great. I want you to check your weight only once a week, or once every two weeks. You should weigh yourself at the same time each day, and you should be in the nude.

Weight fluctuates on a daily basis. You get on the scale after dinner and weigh in three pounds heavier than you did in the morning. A women's weight is worse than a man's as far as fluctuation goes; we have other factors like water weight and hormones. This is why I don't recommend weighing yourself every day. Your change will be more visible in your clothes. Another cool way to track your changes is to set aside a favorite pair of pants and shirt (that don't fit well or are very snug) that you can use as measuring tools. In about three weeks, you should notice some changes, not only in the way your clothes fit, but also in your energy level. After a month or so, you will begin to notice even more changes in your clothes, but results vary from person to person.

I want to see real life-changing habits that can lead to a long, healthy, fit life. Whatever you do, don't forget that training your body needs to be a part of your daily routine.

Room 3
BE FIT NOT FAKE

In this room, I lay out some facts and review some supplements that I think are essential. Flip through and stop when you see something you like. Although I'd like everyone to read it in its entirety, I'm a realist.

Your basic Nutrition Facts food label will include: serving size, servings per container, calories, calories from fat, total fat, cholesterol, sodium, potassium, total carbohydrates, dietary fiber, sugars, and protein. It will also go into what percentages of vitamins are in the food, as well as the ingredients. Ingredients are listed in order from the highest quantity to the least quantity. Therefore, the first ingredient on the label is what the product is mostly made of, and then it trickles downward.

So, starting from the top and working our way down, we will begin with, serving size and servings per container. The size of the serving on the food package influences the number of calories and all the nutrient amounts listed on the top part of the label. **You should pay close attention to the serving size**, especially how many servings there are in the food package. Then ask yourself, "How many servings am I consuming?"(e.g. ½ serving, 1 serving, or more).

In this example, we will use rice. Let's say the package reads 'Serving size 1 cup, servings per container 2'. One serving of rice equals one cup. If you ate the whole package, you would eat **two** cups. That doubles the calories, carbohydrates, fat, and other nutrient numbers, including the

% daily values as shown in the sample label below. The nutrition labels are also based on an individual that is eating 2000 calories a day. Most bodybuilders, and Olympic athletes consume such large quantities as this... hint, hint! You can see how the numbers must be taken into consideration to your personal fitness and health goals.

1

Nutrition Facts

Serving Size 1 cup (228g)
Servings Per Container 2

Amount Per Serving

Calories 250   Calories from Fat 110

	% Daily Value*
Total Fat 12g	**18%**
Saturated Fat 3g	**15%**
Trans Fat 3g	
Cholesterol 30mg	**10%**
Sodium 470mg	**20%**
Total Carbohydrate 31g	**10%**
Dietary Fiber 0g	**0%**
Sugars 5g	
Protein 5g	
Vitamin A	4%
Vitamin C	2%
Calcium	20%
Iron	4%

* Percent Daily Values are based on a 2,000 calorie diet.
Your Daily Values may be higher or lower depending on
your calorie needs.

	Calories:	2,000	2,500
Total Fat	Less than	65g	80g
Sat Fat	Less than	20g	25g
Cholesterol	Less than	300mg	300mg
Sodium	Less than	2,400mg	2,400mg
Total Carbohydrate		300g	375g
Dietary Fiber		25g	30g

Calories provide a measure of how much energy you get
from a serving of this food. Many Americans consume more
calories than they need, without meeting recommended

intakes for a number of nutrients. The calorie section of the label can help you manage your weight (i.e., gain, loss, or maintain.) **Remember: the number of servings you consume determines the number of calories you actually eat (use your portion amount).**

In our example, rice has 250 calories in one serving, and 110 calories from fat. This means almost half the calories from a single serving come from fat. What if you consumed the entire package? You would be consuming two servings, or 500 calories and 220 would come from fat. The nutrients on the labels are also very important. Eating too much **fat, saturated fat, trans fat, cholesterol, or sodium** may increase your risk of certain chronic diseases like heart disease, some cancers, or high blood pressure. Instead, buy products that contain high amounts of dietary fiber, vitamin A, vitamin C, calcium, and iron.

Tip: You don't want to see partially hydrogenated oil, aspartame, or high fructose corn syrup (sugar) in the products that you are purchasing; these products rob us of a healthy, long life.

Every gram of carbohydrate is equal to four calories. If you find yourself having super size French fries at McDonald's, you should think about these little facts. A super size order contains about 77 carbs, you multiple that by four and your calories from carbs are 308. Next, every one gram of protein is also equal to four calories, in the same fries you have 9 grams of proteins, so you multiply that by 4 and you get 36 calories from protein. Finally, every one gram of fat is equal to nine calories; the same size fry has 29 fat grams, multiply this by 9 and you get 261 calories from fat. So, not including saturated fat, your yummy fries have given you 605 calories, and just to think you haven't even had your burger yet! This is really rather disturbing if you think about it.

According to recent results of the National Health and Nutrition Examination Survey (NHANES) 1999 indicate that an estimated 61% of U.S. adults are either overweight or obese. This is not to knock carbohydrates, because we need them to function properly. This example is to help you get a picture of how important it is to be conscious of what you are eating, and how it will affect your body.

Fats

Fats are essential to your diet, and not all fat is bad fat. Fat doesn't necessarily make you fat, but eating more fat than your body needs in a day will definitely contribute to your weight problem. To keep this simple, we will talk about good fat and bad fat, also known as saturated/trans fatty acid/hydrogenated (bad fat) and poly & mono unsaturated (good fats). Bad fats can eventually kill you in the process of making you obese. Bad fats can be found in things like packaged snack foods, fast food french-fries, and margarine. Bad fats can cause heart disease, give you high cholesterol, and may cause heart attacks and strokes over the long haul.

Food in its unprocessed form is needed to energize the body, to assist it in the natural process of self-healing, and natural regulation. The body requires seven basic nutrients for optimal functioning. These nutrients are: carbohydrates, fats, proteins, vitamins, minerals, fiber, and water. We should eat a variety of natural or organic foods to get all nutrients in a sufficient manner. Most American diets are loaded with too much fat, sugar, and salt, which leads to high cholesterol, heart disease, colon cancer, and high blood pressure.

The simple reality is that too many calories, too much fat, and too many unhealthy carbohydrates will cause you to be overweight or obese. Personally, the less meat I eat, the better my gut feels. Once you are equipped with the knowledge on food facts, you are charged to act on this understanding accordingly! In my opinion, obesity in America should be contributed to the following: excess carbohydrates, excess calories, lack of knowledge on what roles food plays in your body, and lack of exercise. Everything in life requires balance. This is why every diet and every routine is so unique to each individual. Eating the foods that I have suggested will allow you to make a plan that works for you.

The key to maintaining a healthy lifestyle is exercise, healthy eating habits, and drinking plenty of water. To fill nutritional gaps and enhance your health conscious efforts, you should support your diet by taking vitamins. Your food does provide nutrients for your body, but you need an extra boost to help sustain a strong body, a focused mind, as well as fight off diseases.

Most people think that they can get the full amount of nutrients they need strictly from food. This is partially true. You can, but you would have to eat totally unprocessed foods, and you would need to eat them in large amounts. In our society, this is rarely achieved. So, your alternative is ... supplementing!

Below, you will find a list of vitamins and supplements that I believe will enhance your life. You don't have to take them all, but at a minimum give a multi-vitamin a try.

Vitamin & Supplements List

Multi-Vitamin - fills nutritional gaps. A whole food-based vitamin is best.

Vitamin C - this vitamin is great for the skin, fighting colds, strengthening joints, and bones. Research has shown that it also combats heart disease and some types of cancer.

B vitamins - are good for assisting the body in processing proteins, increasing mental alertness, and energy.

Vitamin D - helps keep bones healthy and strong. Great for people who spend lots of time in the sun (replacing lost vitamin D).

Calcium/Magnesium - will support strong bones and teeth, increases good heart health. These two products are best when used together.

Chromium - is very helpful in balancing blood sugar, and will assist in cravings in conjunction with a healthy diet.

Coenzyme Q10 - has been noted in medical research as the cure all (in conjunction with a healthy lifestyle of course). This nutrient is a great antioxidant that regulates blood pressure, sustains heart functions, and much more.

Omega 3, 6, & 9 (EFA) - is essential to sustaining cardiovascular health, lowering blood pressure, and cholesterol.

Green Tea/Green Tea Pills - improves the ratios for cholesterol levels, kills headaches, lifts mood, fights fat absorption, and builds up the immune system.

The benefits are unimaginable.

How is everything flowing? I must discuss proper bowel elimination. Many Americans have fallen victim to believing that having a bowel movement every third day is ok, and normal. This is FALSE, FALSE, and FALSE. If you eat three times a day, you should go three times a day... at least once!

No joke, many people are being stricken with unexplained diseases, plagued with headaches, fatigue, and even depression. A simple cleansing may be the answer.

Regularity is basically determined by your current colon health, diet, and lifestyle. If you find that you are constipated often, I recommend staying away from greasy, fatty foods like fries and burgers. Also, limit your candy and other sweet sugary foods. Replace these habits with more fruit and vegetables, and plenty of water. Sometimes, the body may need to be cleansed and detoxified before you can see the full benefits of your new eating habits or exercise routines. The build up of waste in your intestines can begin to spill over into other areas of your body, and this is the beginning of a slew of other health issues. Your pre-requisite to this program can be a colon cleanser, which can be picked up at any local health food store, if necessary.

Quick Tips To Remember

1. Try not to eat after 7:30 pm.
2. Use a smaller plate when making your meals. Using a smaller plate can help trick the eye to make your brain think you have plenty of food on your plate. I know it sounds silly, but it works.
3. Drink lots of water. No alcohol intake. It provides empty calories and empty carbohydrates.
4. Try to take a brief walk after dinner. Don't run back for that second plate of food. Give yourself some time for your brain to tell your stomach you are full. If you are truly hungry after 10-15 minutes of waiting, then have a small helping. Only go back for seconds on vegetables and water! Don't just sit around and wait for the 15 minutes to be over either. Get up, clean the kitchen, talk on the

phone, or walk for 15 minutes. The point is to do something that keeps your mind going, and you won't make food such a priority.

5. Take this journey with a friend if possible.
6. Don't suck down half a soda while you are eating. The stomach acid can't properly digest your food when you put in soda, tea, or coffee. You actually disturb the enzymes that help break down food. If you find that you must have something, opt for water with lemon after you have finished your meal. Adding lemon will help relieve indigestion such as heartburn, bloating, and belching. It also stimulates digestion and elimination.
7. Open your hand... this is a good portion size of protein and carbohydrates to eat. I know you think that is extremely small, but it is all about change, remember! Of course, you can load up your plate with vegetables.
8. If you remove a negative from your life, you must replace it with a positive. Don't just stop eating cookies, replace it with strawberries. Remove and replace... just keep it healthy and positive.

Stay Fit, Stay Alive!

Before doing any workout, you should always warm up for 5-10 minutes. After completing a workout, you should stretch and cool down for 10-15 minutes. Full body toning (you'll see below) should be done two to three times a week, such as a Monday, Wednesday, Friday plan, or Tuesday and Thursday. Cardio should be done 5-7 days a week.

Cardio
You can get your cardiovascular workout in by doing any of the following exercise: jumping jacks, skipping rope, walking in place with light hand-weights, outdoor walking or jogging. If you can afford to get home cardio equipment like a stationary bike, treadmill, or elliptical machine, that would be great. Your cardio goal should be to work out for 30 minutes, and increase this time as you feel strong enough. If this is too much to start with, don't get discouraged, work at your pace for the first week or two, and then continue to increase the time. Remember, make a change in the right direction... a little goes a long way.

Full Body Toning
The Push-up - Lie chest-down with your hands at shoulder level, palms flat on the floor and slightly more than shoulder-width apart, with your feet together and parallel to each other (for beginners, you can start on your knees or leaning against a wall instead of being on the floor). Straighten your arms as you push your body up off the floor. Keep your hands fixed at the same position and keep your body straight. Try not to bend or arch your upper or lower back as you push up. Exhale

as your arms straighten out. Pause and then lower your body towards the floor by bending your arms. Lower until your chest touches the floor, pause, and repeat sequence. What I love about the push-up is that it engages all of your upper torso muscles. Push-ups are the best!

Triceps Kickbacks- Stand center and hold a weight in the right hand. Bend torso forward, keeping back flat (like a table top) and keep abs pulled in, and rest left elbow on the knee for support. Pull the arm up next to your rib cage, elbow bent, and straighten the arm out behind you, squeezing the back of your arm without moving the elbow. Lower back down and repeat. Then switch to the other arm.

Bicep Hammer Curls- Stand with feet hip-width apart, and hold dumb-bells at sides, palms facing the thighs. Bend the elbows and bring the weight towards the shoulders in a bicep curl, taking care not to move the elbows away from your sides. Lower your back down (but keep the tension by not relaxing all the way) and repeat. These curls allow you to train the forearm at the same time as the bicep.

Lunges (working your lower body) - Stand in a split stance, right leg in front, left leg in back. (You can use weights for added tension), bend both knees and lower into a lunge, keeping front knee BEHIND the toe and knees, no lower than 90 degree angles. Squeeze through the heel to lift back up.

Belly Bicycles (abs) - Lie face up with lower back pressed to the floor. Cradle head in your hands, elbows out, and bend right knee, pulling it towards your chest while touching the knee with the opposite elbow. Begin a slow pedal motion by touching opposite elbow to opposite knee, alternating each side. Keep the abs pulled in and breathe.

Belly Buster (abs) - Lie face up with legs crossed straight in the air (feet to the ceiling). Place finger tips on side of head near temple area or cross arms on chest, and lift your upper torso, pause, and return to floor and repeat. In this same position (after you've completed a few sets of the above), hold upper torso up and lift buttocks from floor using your lower abdominal muscles.

You will be able to feel a difference in your body as well as your mind once you begin working out. You will notice that you think clearer and have more energy. No more sluggish, foggy thinking!

Calories, Carbs, Fats, Proteins & Your Weight

When calculating each meal, I balance out the allowed amount of nutrients in each category to create a healthy balance to help achieve top-notch health, energy, and weight goals. This may vary based on the individual. Variations can be lowered to speed up weight loss, or even raised for competitive athletes and body builders. To begin, you will need to determine how many calories you should intake each day. The 2000-calorie diet requirements that you see listed everywhere is very generic. Your calories requirements can fluctuate based on your height, age, weight, and daily activity levels. Understanding where your calories are coming from will help you to make wiser choices.

Calories are made up of carbohydrates, fats, and protein. Carbohydrates contain 4 calories per gram. Proteins contain 4 calories per gram, and fat contains 9 calories per gram. You can see just from that little breakdown how too much fat can impact your weight loss efforts. Now, one pound is equivalent to 3500 calories, so to lose one pound a week, you need to reduce your caloric intake by 3500 calories a week. If your normal routine has been eating 2000 calories a day, you need to reduce that to 1500 calories per day. This can be done through a simple diet change. Combined with exercise, you will have quicker, easier results. I don't want you eating 1500 calories of junk food though. You need to replace the overindulgence on high fat, high carbohydrate foods with a more balanced approach to eating. I have given you the tools, now it's up to you to use them.

Weight and Height Chart

Below, you will find general guidelines in weight/height for each gender. Remember, these are ranges that have not taken into consideration your actual body fat percentages, or genetic dispositions.

The height is measured without shoes, and the weight is without clothes.

	WEIGHT FOR HEIGHT TABLE	
HEIGHT	MEN	WOMEN
4'10	⇒	92-121
4'11	⇒	95-124
5'0	⇒	98-127
5'1	105-134	101-130
5'2	108-137	104-134
5'3	111-141	107-138
5'4	114-145	110-142
5'5	117-149	114-146
5'6	121-154	118-150
5'7	125-159	122-154

5'8	129-16.93	126-159
5'9	133-16.97	130-16.94
5'10	137-172	134-16.99
5'11	141-177	138-173
6'0	145-182	142-177
6'1	149-187	146-181
6'2	153-192	150-185
6'3	157-196	154-189

When using this chart for women 18-25 years old, subtract 1 pound for each year under 25.

HEALTH INFORMATION YOU SHOULD KNOW

[2] Did you know, according to the National Center for Health Statistics that an estimated 16% of children and adolescents aged 6-19 years are overweight? (http://www.cdc.gov/nchs/) [According to the results from the 1999-2002 National Health and Nutrition Examination Survey (NHANES), using measured heights and weights] This represents a 45% increase from the 1988-1994 estimates obtained from NHANES III. This tells us that we are now infecting the next generation with obesity, and a higher risk for high blood pressure, stroke, diabetes, and even heart disease. Poor eating habits will inevitably increase a person's risk of cancer and other chronic health disease (Center for Disease Control and Prevention).

The food we put in our mouth feeds our cells. Our choice of food can allow the cells to flourish or be destroyed. Destroying those cells causes increased episodes of illness. Research shows that the causes of many diseases are 50% genetics and 50% the food you eat.

The idea in consuming foods should be to get as close to

natural, wholesome foods as possible.

I would like to briefly discuss the dangers of an ingredient that is found in just about all shelf foods. The FDA has also gotten involved in ridding our food products of this ingredient, once the severities of its effect were fully evaluated. The product is known as Trans Fats. [3]According to the FDA, trans fats are made when manufacturers add hydrogen to vegetable oil - a process called hydrogenation. Hydrogenation increases the shelf life and flavoring of foods containing these fats.

Trans fats attach to your cell walls, and eventually, your arteries. Consuming foods with partially hydrogenated oil in the ingredients list can lead to disease and obesity. If you consume large amounts of saturated fat, you will be fat.

Trans fat can be found in vegetable shortenings, margarine, crackers, cookies, snack foods, and other foods made with or fried in partially hydrogenated oils. Trans fat, like saturated fat and dietary cholesterol, raises the LDL cholesterol that increases your risk for coronary heart disease. Americans consume on average 4 to 5 times as much saturated fat as Trans fat in their diets.

Below are lists that identify foods that may contain unhealthy fats (Trans fats or partially hydrogenated oils), and a list of foods that usually do not contain partially hydrogenated oils. You should always read the labels for accuracy.

4

Foods Commonly Containing Partially Hydrogenated Oils

Cake mixes, biscuit, pancake and cornbread mixes, frostings
Cakes, cookies, muffins, pies, donuts
Crackers
Peanut butter (except fresh-ground)
Frozen entrees and meals
Frozen bakery products, toaster pastries, waffles, pancakes
Most prepared frozen meats and fish (such as fish sticks)
In-organic French fries
Whipped toppings
Margarines, shortening
Instant mashed potatoes
Taco shells
Cocoa mix
Microwave popcorn

Many Brands of these Foods May Contain Partially Hydrogenated Oils

(Check the labels!)
Breakfast cereals
Corn chips, potato chips
Frozen pizza, frozen burritos, most frozen snack foods
Low-fat ice creams
Noodle soup cups
Bread
Pasta mixes
Sauce mixes

Foods that usually do not contain Partially Hydrogenated Oils
All fruits and vegetables
Dairy products, including cheese and some ice creams
Meat, poultry, fish
Sugar, flour
Spices, condiments, pickles, salad dressings, and mayonnaise
Jams and jellies
Beans, grains, nuts and seeds
Plain popcorn (not microwave)
Pretzels, rice crackers
Coffee & tea
Frozen fruits & vegetables
Canned fruits & vegetables
Organic Products

The next ingredient to eliminate from you diet is aspartame. This ingredient can be found in diet drinks, certain gums, many products that claim to be sugar-free, artificial sweeteners, and many more. I must reiterate that it is very important to read the ingredient labels. I encourage you to eliminate this product from your diet. Slower may be easier than going cold turkey. There is a possibility of having headaches from the initial withdrawal symptoms. I did some research and found several startling facts about aspartame. Diet drinks were once a life-saver for me, but with dedication to change, I shook the habit. Here are some of the killer facts I have learned about aspartame:

- [5] Aspartame is a brain drug that stimulates your brain so you think that the food you're eating tastes sweet. If you pay attention, you'll notice that when using Aspartame, everything you eat at the same time also tastes sweet! This may be why aspartame causes you to crave carbohydrates. Hence, you won't lose weight using it.

- Aspartame's 40% Aspartic Acid is an "excitotoxin" in the brain and excites neurons to death, i.e. it kills brain cells and causes other nerve damage.
- Aspartame triggers migraine headaches. The Usenet is filled with posts by people who have pinned their migraines down to aspartame consumption.
- Aspartames breakdown products attack the body's tissues and create formaldehyde, which builds up in the tissues forever. Remember the smelly, eye-watering fumes from the frogs you dissected in school? They were preserved with formaldehyde! Formaldehyde is thought to cause cancer.
- Aspartame also breaks down to diketopiperazine [DKP], which is proven to cause brain tumors!

As you can see, some supplements aren't worth the risk!

Room 4
Make It Happen

This room is fun. You will find plenty of tools that will assist you in becoming a Bloggers Diet success story. Blog often, email me your questions, and enjoy the process!

Below is a guide on how to feel bloated, fatigued, and pack on the pounds. Simply consume these products, don't exercise, and you will be well on your way.

FAST FAT

Fast Food Deterrent:

Places	Calories	Carbohydrates	Fats
Burger King Whopper	680	53	39
McDonald's Big Mac	590	47	34
McDonald's Shake	360	59	9
Pizza Hut (1 slice Med Pepperoni)	280	28	14
Taco Bell (1 Steak Chalupa Baja)	400	27	24

Wendy's Med Fries	420	55	20
KFC Original Breast	400	16.9	24
Captain D's Broiled Fish Platter	735	131	7
Carvel Regular Choco	420	48	22

Let's see what it takes to burn calories:

The following figures are estimated on a 150lb-person working out for at least one hour at the activity.

- Bicycling - <10mph - 265 calories burned in 1 hour.
- Cleaning house vigorously - 300 calories burned in 1 hour.
- Running - 5mph (12-min mile) - 563 calories burned in 1 hour.
- Swimming for fun - 400 calories burned in 1 hour.
- Walking 2 mph (slow pace) - 16.90 calories burned in 1 hour.
- Walking 3.5mph, uphill - 400 calories burned in 1 hour.
- Weightlifting, vigorous effort - 400 calories burned per 1 hour.

Recipes: Breakfast

- Oatmeal with cinnamon (no milk or butter), berries on side.
- Protein shake with banana or berries.
- 2 boiled eggs, slice of whole grain bread, and mango slice.
- Vegetable omelet with fruit on side.
- Salmon, with your choice of veggies.
- Scrambled eggs, turkey bacon, and fruit.
- Turkey sausage, whole grain bread, and lettuce or spinach.
- Yogurt with fruit, and handful of granola.
- Cottage cheese, pineapples, and a boiled egg.
- Bran cereal or whole grain cereal, fat free milk, and fruit.

Lunch

- Pita with lean meat and vegetables.
- Green salad with chicken breast, turkey, or fish.
- Broccoli with brown rice and your choice of protein.
- Black beans with brown rice and green vegetables.
- Chicken or turkey breast with leaf spinach.

Dinner

- Turkey or chicken breast, sweet potato, and a green salad.
- Lamb or any lean meat, green beans, and salad.
- Wild rice, salad, salmon, or any lean meat.
- Chicken salad.

Feel free to mix and match meals. Learn new recipes, but keep the same basic, simple-to-follow principles. These principles are to eat complex carbohydrates like sweet potato, brown rice, red potatoes, on occasion. Consume lots of green foods and vegetables; consume lean protein, preferably organic meat. Stay away from processed and packaged foods. Stay clear of white flour, white sugar, fast food, and food that contain trans fats. Drink lots of water, take necessary supplements, exercise, and enjoy life.

FAQ

Q. Do I have to work out every day?

A. If you are just beginning a fitness routine, I recommend working out a minimum of three times per week. The goal would be to build up to five to six times a week. Your workout does not have to be long either. I can develop plans that are 30 to 60 minutes, and cover the entire body.

Q. Is it true that I can sleep off my weight?

A. I wish this were true... Sleep is a component in weight loss. It is ideal to get seven or more hours of sleep per night. Sleep allows your body to de-stress, and your body to replenish itself from all the demands that we place on it during our waking hours. The less sleep you get, the more damage you render to your health.

Q. I am considering acupuncture for weight loss. What is your take on this?

A. Acupuncture is a traditional Chinese therapy. It has been used to treat many aliments. As with any alternative therapy, it takes some change on the part of the patient to see maximum benefits. I recommend also changing your view on food and fitness while trying acupuncture for weight loss.

Q. My girlfriend wants me to try hypnosis for my bulging belly. Will this make me lose weight?

A. Hypnosis performed by a certified therapist can be useful in weight loss if the person is open to the suggestions made by the therapist, and has a strong desire to change basic eating patterns.

Q. I have many business meetings. I cannot always take a lunch. What should I order at a restaurant?

A. This is a question that I get all the time. With so many different diets around, a person can get bogged down and simply give up on trying to be a conscious eater.
Here are the tips I normally recommend: Always choose white meat not red (go for fish, turkey or chicken). Go for baked or grilled not fried or battered. Always select a salad, and do not use a creamy dressing. Go for Italian or some form of vinaigrette. Do not bother eating the buttered bread, French fries, ketchup, or mayo. If the restaurant offers vegetables, definitely order a serving of them. Always choose water or unsweetened tea. Pass on the sugary, empty calorie sodas.

Q. How long will it take to see results from the Bloggers Diet?

A. Results will vary based on the person's level of fitness upon starting. With this in mind, the average person can see results within the first week when working from Room 2, and immediate changes can be felt when working in Room 1. I develop personal plans for individuals based on their personality & lifestyle. These plans yield very favorable results.

Q. Is this just another FAD diet?

A. There is nothing faddish about Bloggers Diet. It takes the essence of human nature, and nurtures the positive while eliminating the negative. I do not just want you to stop eating processed food. I want you to know why you are changing, tell me how you feel about the change, vent when you struggle with the change, and replace the poison food with life sustaining alternatives.

Q. I just need to flatten my tummy. What targeting fitness should I do?

A. I wish it were so simple. The best way to flatten your tummy is to do 30 to 45 minutes of cardio, incorporate a good fat burner, and eat lots of vegetable s and lean proteins. Once you have begun this regimen, you can begin doing various abdominal exercise like crunches, bicycles, and so forth.

7-Day Quick start meal ideas

DAY 1

Breakfast:
¾ cup Kashi Cereal with ½-cup soy, rice or almond milk
Protein shake or two eggs
20 oz water and 8 oz green or black tea (no sugar)

Lunch:
Mixed greens salad with healthy fixings, no creamy dressing.
Add chopped turkey or chicken breast
20 oz of water and 8 oz green tea

Dinner:
Grilled salmon
Lemon broccoli
Side salad
20 oz Water

Snack options (2 per day):
Protein shake
Hummus on celery
Peanut or almond butter on an apple
Turkey roll up

DAY 2

Breakfast:
1-cup oatmeal (not instant) with cinnamon & nuts

Protein shake or two eggs
20 oz water and 8 oz of green or black tea

Lunch:
¾ cups black beans
1 piece chicken breast
Mixed green salads
20 oz water and 8 oz green tea

Dinner:
Mixed greens salad with healthy fixings, no creamy dressing.
Chicken breast
Sweet potato
20 oz water

Snack options (2 per day):
Protein shake
Hummus on celery
Peanut or almond butter on an apple
Turkey roll up

DAY 3

Breakfast:
Omelet, salsa
1 slice whole grain bread
20 oz water and 8 oz green or black tea

Lunch:
Pita with turkey breast, mixed lettuce, tomatoes, and hummus
Carrot sticks

20 oz water and 8 oz green tea

Dinner:
Baked chicken
½ cup brown rice
Assorted veggies
20 oz water

Snack options (2 per day):
Protein shake
Hummus on celery
Peanut or almond butter on an apple
Turkey roll up

DAY 4

Breakfast:
Protein smoothie
20 oz water

Lunch:
Tilapia
Mixed green salad
½ cup brown rice
20 oz water and 8 oz of green tea

Dinner:
Tuna
½ cup brown rice
Mixed veggies
20 oz water

Snack options (2 per day):
Protein shake
Hummus on celery
Peanut or almond butter on an apple
Turkey roll up

DAY 5

Breakfast:
¾ cup Kashi Cereal with ½-cup soy, rice or almond milk
Protein shake or two eggs
20 oz water and 8 oz green or black tea (no sugar)

Lunch:
Mixed greens salad with healthy fixings, no creamy dressing.
Add chopped turkey or chicken breast
20 oz of water and 8 oz green tea

Dinner:
Grilled salmon
Lemon broccoli
Side Salad
20 oz Water

Snack options (2 per day):
Protein Shake
Hummus on celery
Peanut or almond butter on an apple
Turkey roll up

DAY 6

Breakfast:
1-cup oatmeal (not instant) with cinnamon & nuts
Protein shake or two eggs
20 oz water and 8 oz of green or black tea

Lunch:
¾ cups black beans
1 piece chicken breast
Mixed green salads
20 oz water and 8 oz green tea

Dinner:
Mixed greens salad with healthy fixings, no creamy dressing.
Chicken breast
Sweet potato
20 oz water

Snack options (2 per day):
Protein shake
Hummus on celery
Peanut or almond butter on an apple
Turkey roll up

DAY 7

Breakfast:
Omelet, salsa
1 slice whole grain bread
 20 oz water and 8 oz green or black tea

Lunch:

Pita with turkey breast, mixed lettuce, tomatoes, and hummus
Carrot sticks
20 oz water and 8 oz green tea

Dinner:
Baked chicken
½ cup brown rice
Assorted veggies
20 oz water

Snack options (2 per day):
Protein shake
Hummus on celery
Peanut or almond butter on an apple
Turkey roll up

References:
Room 3

1. "How to Understand and Use the Nutrition Facts Label",
   U.S. Food and Drug Administration/June 2000,
   http://www.cfsan.fda.gov/~dms/foodlab.html
2. National Health Statistics-http://www.cdc.gov/nchs/
3. "Q & A about Trans Fats", U.S. Food and Drug
   Administration/June 2003,
   http://www.cfsan.fda.gov/~dms/qatrans2.html
4. "Trans fatty acids",
   http://www.recoverymedicine.com/hydrogenated_oil_contai
   ning_foods.html
5. "Is diet coke bad for you",
   http://joi.ito.com/archives/2002/10/26/is_diet_coke_bad_for
   _you.html

Expressions

I am glad to be typing this section. It means that the preparation for this project is now complete, and the journey now begins. I want to thank my Lord and Savior Jesus Christ, who gave me forgiveness, focus, vision, and strength. Without Him, I am nothing... with Him I can conquer all things. Thank you for giving me the opportunity to grow into a wise woman of your calling.

Ramon, thank you for continuously motivating me, challenging me, inspiring me, and loving me just for me. You are everything to me, and words can never express the feelings of my heart, but I LOVE YOU... Infinitely!

Victoria, Kimberly, Trinity, and Audrey -Thank you for loving Mama even though she was busy at times typing away. You angels are pure blessings from the hand of God.

Thomas & Annie Tillman (Momma & Bigdaddy) -Thank you for believing in me. Thank you for sacrificing your life to raise me in the fear & admonition of the Lord. I hope to one day repay you in more than words. You are great examples of the power of praying parents.

Wanda (Mommie) & Paul Lee (Daddy) -I love you both. You each hold a special place in my heart. I am a combined expression of all that is good within you...Thank you for giving me life. In loving memory of my mother, Wanda Denise Tillman-Harville, who returned to Heaven on February 7, 2008. I finally finished my book. I love you!

Josefa Tangui (Mom) - Thank you for raising such a well-rounded son, for all your inspiration, and your guided thinking.

To everyone reading, please remember in all that you do... You choose your circumstances, so choose wisely!

Life is short, tomorrow is promised to no one. So get healthy, love others, and show gratitude to our Creator!

Nakisha R. Guzman

www.ingramcontent.com/pod-product-compliance
Lightning Source LLC
Chambersburg PA
CBHW031203270326
41931CB00006B/383